ATS-38   ADMISSION TEST SERIES

This is your
PASSBOOK for...

Certified Electronic Technician (CET)

Test Preparation Study Guide
Questions & Answers

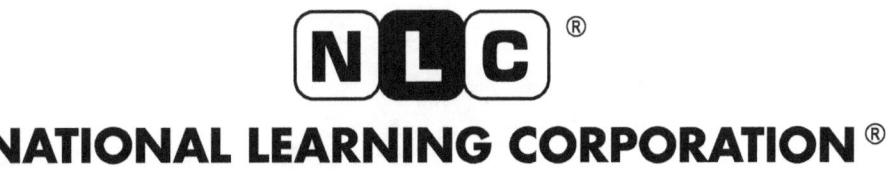

NATIONAL LEARNING CORPORATION®

COPYRIGHT NOTICE

This book is SOLELY intended for, is sold ONLY to, and its use is RESTRICTED to individual, bona fide applicants or candidates who qualify by virtue of having seriously filed applications for appropriate license, certificate, professional and/or promotional advancement, higher school matriculation, scholarship, or other legitimate requirements of education and/or governmental authorities.

This book is NOT intended for use, class instruction, tutoring, training, duplication, copying, reprinting, excerption, or adaptation, etc., by:

1) Other publishers
2) Proprietors and/or Instructors of "Coaching" and/or Preparatory Courses
3) Personnel and/or Training Divisions of commercial, industrial, and governmental organizations
4) Schools, colleges, or universities and/or their departments and staffs, including teachers and other personnel
5) Testing Agencies or Bureaus
6) Study groups which seek by the purchase of a single volume to copy and/or duplicate and/or adapt this material for use by the group as a whole without having purchased individual volumes for each of the members of the group
7) Et al.

Such persons would be in violation of appropriate Federal and State statutes.

PROVISION OF LICENSING AGREEMENTS – Recognized educational, commercial, industrial, and governmental institutions and organizations, and others legitimately engaged in educational pursuits, including training, testing, and measurement activities, may address request for a licensing agreement to the copyright owners, who will determine whether, and under what conditions, including fees and charges, the materials in this book may be used them. In other words, a licensing facility exists for the legitimate use of the material in this book on other than an individual basis. However, it is asseverated and affirmed here that the material in this book CANNOT be used without the receipt of the express permission of such a licensing agreement from the Publishers. Inquiries re licensing should be addressed to the company, attention rights and permissions department.

All rights reserved, including the right of reproduction in whole or in part, in any form or by any means, electronic or mechanical, including photocopying, recording, or by any information storage and retrieval system, without permission in writing from the Publisher.

Copyright © 2024 by
National Learning Corporation

212 Michael Drive, Syosset, NY 11791
(516) 921-8888 • www.passbooks.com
E-mail: info@passbooks.com

PUBLISHED IN THE UNITED STATES OF AMERICA

PASSBOOK® SERIES

THE *PASSBOOK® SERIES* has been created to prepare applicants and candidates for the ultimate academic battlefield – the examination room.

At some time in our lives, each and every one of us may be required to take an examination – for validation, matriculation, admission, qualification, registration, certification, or licensure.

Based on the assumption that every applicant or candidate has met the basic formal educational standards, has taken the required number of courses, and read the necessary texts, the *PASSBOOK® SERIES* furnishes the one special preparation which may assure passing with confidence, instead of failing with insecurity. Examination questions – together with answers – are furnished as the basic vehicle for study so that the mysteries of the examination and its compounding difficulties may be eliminated or diminished by a sure method.

This book is meant to help you pass your examination provided that you qualify and are serious in your objective.

The entire field is reviewed through the huge store of content information which is succinctly presented through a provocative and challenging approach – the question-and-answer method.

A climate of success is established by furnishing the correct answers at the end of each test.

You soon learn to recognize types of questions, forms of questions, and patterns of questioning. You may even begin to anticipate expected outcomes.

You perceive that many questions are repeated or adapted so that you can gain acute insights, which may enable you to score many sure points.

You learn how to confront new questions, or types of questions, and to attack them confidently and work out the correct answers.

You note objectives and emphases, and recognize pitfalls and dangers, so that you may make positive educational adjustments.

Moreover, you are kept fully informed in relation to new concepts, methods, practices, and directions in the field.

You discover that you are actually taking the examination all the time: you are preparing for the examination by "taking" an examination, not by reading extraneous and/or supererogatory textbooks.

In short, this PASSBOOK®, used directedly, should be an important factor in helping you to pass your test.

CERTIFIED ELECTRONIC TECHNICIAN

Since 1966, the National Electronic Association has sponsored a certification program to provide recognition for qualified technicians, and issues, upon passing a written examination, a certificate recognized around the world as evidence of proficiency and qualification in electronics.

These Certified Electronic Technicians then become eligible to join the International Society of Certified Electronic Technicians (ISCET).

To become a CET, a candidate must have at least four years' experience in electronic servicing and must pass a rigorous examination in electronics.

This book is intended to provide the candidate with sample study examinations of the type and in the areas given in the Certified Electronic Technician examination. The editors are confident that study of this book, along with the requisite knowledge and experience in the electronic field, will lead to success on the examination.

HOW TO TAKE A TEST

You have studied long, hard and conscientiously.

With your official admission card in hand, and your heart pounding, you have been admitted to the examination room.

You note that there are several hundred other applicants in the examination room waiting to take the same test.

They all appear to be equally well prepared.

You know that nothing but your best effort will suffice. The "moment of truth" is at hand: you now have to demonstrate objectively, in writing, your knowledge of content and your understanding of subject matter.

You are fighting the most important battle of your life—to pass and/or score high on an examination which will determine your career and provide the economic basis for your livelihood.

What extra, special things should you know and should you do in taking the examination?

I. YOU MUST PASS AN EXAMINATION

A. WHAT EVERY CANDIDATE SHOULD KNOW
   Examination applicants often ask us for help in preparing for the written test. What can I study in advance? What kinds of questions will be asked? How will the test be given? How will the papers be graded?

B. HOW ARE EXAMS DEVELOPED?
   Examinations are carefully written by trained technicians who are specialists in the field known as "psychological measurement," in consultation with recognized authorities in the field of work that the test will cover. These experts recommend the subject matter areas or skills to be tested; only those knowledges or skills important to your success on the job are included. The most reliable books and source materials available are used as references. Together, the experts and technicians judge the difficulty level of the questions.
   Test technicians know how to phrase questions so that the problem is clearly stated. Their ethics do not permit "trick" or "catch" questions. Questions may have been tried out on sample groups, or subjected to statistical analysis, to determine their usefulness.
   Written tests are often used in combination with performance tests, ratings of training and experience, and oral interviews. All of these measures combine to form the best-known means of finding the right person for the right job.

II. HOW TO PASS THE WRITTEN TEST

A. BASIC STEPS

1) Study the announcement

How, then, can you know what subjects to study? Our best answer is: "Learn as much as possible about the class of positions for which you've applied." The exam will test the knowledge, skills and abilities needed to do the work.

Your most valuable source of information about the position you want is the official exam announcement. This announcement lists the training and experience qualifications. Check these standards and apply only if you come reasonably close to meeting them. Many jurisdictions preview the written test in the exam announcement by including a section called "Knowledge and Abilities Required," "Scope of the Examination," or some similar heading. Here you will find out specifically what fields will be tested.

2) Choose appropriate study materials

If the position for which you are applying is technical or advanced, you will read more advanced, specialized material. If you are already familiar with the basic principles of your field, elementary textbooks would waste your time. Concentrate on advanced textbooks and technical periodicals. Think through the concepts and review difficult problems in your field.

These are all general sources. You can get more ideas on your own initiative, following these leads. For example, training manuals and publications of the government agency which employs workers in your field can be useful, particularly for technical and professional positions. A letter or visit to the government department involved may result in more specific study suggestions, and certainly will provide you with a more definite idea of the exact nature of the position you are seeking.

3) Study this book!

III. KINDS OF TESTS

Tests are used for purposes other than measuring knowledge and ability to perform specified duties. For some positions, it is equally important to test ability to make adjustments to new situations or to profit from training. In others, basic mental abilities not dependent on information are essential. Questions which test these things may not appear as pertinent to the duties of the position as those which test for knowledge and information. Yet they are often highly important parts of a fair examination. For very general questions, it is almost impossible to help you direct your study efforts. What we can do is to point out some of the more common of these general abilities needed in public service positions and describe some typical questions.

1) General information

Broad, general information has been found useful for predicting job success in some kinds of work. This is tested in a variety of ways, from vocabulary lists to questions about current events. Basic background in some field of work, such as sociology or economics, may be sampled in a group of questions. Often these are principles which have become familiar to most persons through exposure rather than through formal training. It is difficult to advise you how to study for these questions; being alert to the world around you is our best suggestion.

2) Verbal ability

An example of an ability needed in many positions is verbal or language ability. Verbal ability is, in brief, the ability to use and understand words. Vocabulary and grammar tests are typical measures of this ability. Reading comprehension or paragraph interpretation questions are common in many kinds of civil service tests. You are given a paragraph of written material and asked to find its central meaning.

IV. KINDS OF QUESTIONS

1. Multiple-choice Questions

Most popular of the short-answer questions is the "multiple choice" or "best answer" question. It can be used, for example, to test for factual knowledge, ability to solve problems or judgment in meeting situations found at work.

A multiple-choice question is normally one of three types:
- It can begin with an incomplete statement followed by several possible endings. You are to find the one ending which best completes the statement, although some of the others may not be entirely wrong.
- It can also be a complete statement in the form of a question which is answered by choosing one of the statements listed.
- It can be in the form of a problem – again you select the best answer.

Here is an example of a multiple-choice question with a discussion which should give you some clues as to the method for choosing the right answer:

When an employee has a complaint about his assignment, the action which will best help him overcome his difficulty is to
- A. discuss his difficulty with his coworkers
- B. take the problem to the head of the organization
- C. take the problem to the person who gave him the assignment
- D. say nothing to anyone about his complaint

In answering this question, you should study each of the choices to find which is best. Consider choice "A" – Certainly an employee may discuss his complaint with fellow employees, but no change or improvement can result, and the complaint remains unresolved. Choice "B" is a poor choice since the head of the organization probably does not know what assignment you have been given, and taking your problem to him is known as "going over the head" of the supervisor. The supervisor, or person who made the assignment, is the person who can clarify it or correct any injustice. Choice "C" is, therefore, correct. To say nothing, as in choice "D," is unwise. Supervisors have and interest in knowing the problems employees are facing, and the employee is seeking a solution to his problem.

2. True/False

3. Matching Questions

Matching an answer from a column of choices within another column.

V. RECORDING YOUR ANSWERS

Computer terminals are used more and more today for many different kinds of exams.

For an examination with very few applicants, you may be told to record your answers in the test booklet itself. Separate answer sheets are much more common. If this separate answer sheet is to be scored by machine – and this is often the case – it is highly important that you mark your answers correctly in order to get credit.

VI. BEFORE THE TEST

YOUR PHYSICAL CONDITION IS IMPORTANT

If you are not well, you can't do your best work on tests. If you are half asleep, you can't do your best either. Here are some tips:

1) Get about the same amount of sleep you usually get. Don't stay up all night before the test, either partying or worrying—DON'T DO IT!
2) If you wear glasses, be sure to wear them when you go to take the test. This goes for hearing aids, too.
3) If you have any physical problems that may keep you from doing your best, be sure to tell the person giving the test. If you are sick or in poor health, you relay cannot do your best on any test. You can always come back and take the test some other time.

Common sense will help you find procedures to follow to get ready for an examination. Too many of us, however, overlook these sensible measures. Indeed, nervousness and fatigue have been found to be the most serious reasons why applicants fail to do their best on civil service tests. Here is a list of reminders:

- Begin your preparation early – Don't wait until the last minute to go scurrying around for books and materials or to find out what the position is all about.
- Prepare continuously – An hour a night for a week is better than an all-night cram session. This has been definitely established. What is more, a night a week for a month will return better dividends than crowding your study into a shorter period of time.
- Locate the place of the exam – You have been sent a notice telling you when and where to report for the examination. If the location is in a different town or otherwise unfamiliar to you, it would be well to inquire the best route and learn something about the building.
- Relax the night before the test – Allow your mind to rest. Do not study at all that night. Plan some mild recreation or diversion; then go to bed early and get a good night's sleep.
- Get up early enough to make a leisurely trip to the place for the test – This way unforeseen events, traffic snarls, unfamiliar buildings, etc. will not upset you.
- Dress comfortably – A written test is not a fashion show. You will be known by number and not by name, so wear something comfortable.
- Leave excess paraphernalia at home – Shopping bags and odd bundles will get in your way. You need bring only the items mentioned in the official notice you received; usually everything you need is provided. Do not bring reference books to the exam. They will only confuse those last minutes and be taken away from you when in the test room.

- Arrive somewhat ahead of time – If because of transportation schedules you must get there very early, bring a newspaper or magazine to take your mind off yourself while waiting.
- Locate the examination room – When you have found the proper room, you will be directed to the seat or part of the room where you will sit. Sometimes you are given a sheet of instructions to read while you are waiting. Do not fill out any forms until you are told to do so; just read them and be prepared.
- Relax and prepare to listen to the instructions
- If you have any physical problem that may keep you from doing your best, be sure to tell the test administrator. If you are sick or in poor health, you really cannot do your best on the exam. You can come back and take the test some other time.

VII. AT THE TEST

The day of the test is here and you have the test booklet in your hand. The temptation to get going is very strong. Caution! There is more to success than knowing the right answers. You must know how to identify your papers and understand variations in the type of short-answer question used in this particular examination. Follow these suggestions for maximum results from your efforts:

1) Cooperate with the monitor
   The test administrator has a duty to create a situation in which you can be as much at ease as possible. He will give instructions, tell you when to begin, check to see that you are marking your answer sheet correctly, and so on. He is not there to guard you, although he will see that your competitors do not take unfair advantage. He wants to help you do your best.

2) Listen to all instructions
   Don't jump the gun! Wait until you understand all directions. In most civil service tests you get more time than you need to answer the questions. So don't be in a hurry. Read each word of instructions until you clearly understand the meaning. Study the examples, listen to all announcements and follow directions. Ask questions if you do not understand what to do.

3) Identify your papers
   Civil service exams are usually identified by number only. You will be assigned a number; you must not put your name on your test papers. Be sure to copy your number correctly. Since more than one exam may be given, copy your exact examination title.

4) Plan your time
   Unless you are told that a test is a "speed" or "rate of work" test, speed itself is usually not important. Time enough to answer all the questions will be provided, but this does not mean that you have all day. An overall time limit has been set. Divide the total time (in minutes) by the number of questions to determine the approximate time you have for each question.

5) Do not linger over difficult questions
   If you come across a difficult question, mark it with a paper clip (useful to have along) and come back to it when you have been through the booklet. One caution if you do this – be sure to skip a number on your answer sheet as well. Check often to be sure that

you have not lost your place and that you are marking in the row numbered the same as the question you are answering.

6) Read the questions

Be sure you know what the question asks! Many capable people are unsuccessful because they failed to read the questions correctly.

7) Answer all questions

Unless you have been instructed that a penalty will be deducted for incorrect answers, it is better to guess than to omit a question.

8) Speed tests

It is often better NOT to guess on speed tests. It has been found that on timed tests people are tempted to spend the last few seconds before time is called in marking answers at random – without even reading them – in the hope of picking up a few extra points. To discourage this practice, the instructions may warn you that your score will be "corrected" for guessing. That is, a penalty will be applied. The incorrect answers will be deducted from the correct ones, or some other penalty formula will be used.

9) Review your answers

If you finish before time is called, go back to the questions you guessed or omitted to give them further thought. Review other answers if you have time.

10) Return your test materials

If you are ready to leave before others have finished or time is called, take ALL your materials to the monitor and leave quietly. Never take any test material with you. The monitor can discover whose papers are not complete, and taking a test booklet may be grounds for disqualification.

VIII. EXAMINATION TECHNIQUES

1) Read the general instructions carefully. These are usually printed on the first page of the exam booklet. As a rule, these instructions refer to the timing of the examination; the fact that you should not start work until the signal and must stop work at a signal, etc. If there are any special instructions, such as a choice of questions to be answered, make sure that you note this instruction carefully.

2) When you are ready to start work on the examination, that is as soon as the signal has been given, read the instructions to each question booklet, underline any key words or phrases, such as least, best, outline, describe and the like. In this way you will tend to answer as requested rather than discover on reviewing your paper that you listed without describing, that you selected the worst choice rather than the best choice, etc.

3) If the examination is of the objective or multiple-choice type – that is, each question will also give a series of possible answers: A, B, C or D, and you are called upon to select the best answer and write the letter next to that answer on your answer paper – it is advisable to start answering each question in turn. There may be anywhere from 50 to 100 such questions in the three or four hours allotted and you can see how much time would be taken if you read through all the questions before beginning to answer any. Furthermore, if you

come across a question or group of questions which you know would be difficult to answer, it would undoubtedly affect your handling of all the other questions.

4) If the examination is of the essay type and contains but a few questions, it is a moot point as to whether you should read all the questions before starting to answer any one. Of course, if you are given a choice – say five out of seven and the like – then it is essential to read all the questions so you can eliminate the two that are most difficult. If, however, you are asked to answer all the questions, there may be danger in trying to answer the easiest one first because you may find that you will spend too much time on it. The best technique is to answer the first question, then proceed to the second, etc.

5) Time your answers. Before the exam begins, write down the time it started, then add the time allowed for the examination and write down the time it must be completed, then divide the time available somewhat as follows:
   - If 3-1/2 hours are allowed, that would be 210 minutes. If you have 80 objective-type questions, that would be an average of 2-1/2 minutes per question. Allow yourself no more than 2 minutes per question, or a total of 160 minutes, which will permit about 50 minutes to review.
   - If for the time allotment of 210 minutes there are 7 essay questions to answer, that would average about 30 minutes a question. Give yourself only 25 minutes per question so that you have about 35 minutes to review.

6) The most important instruction is to read each question and make sure you know what is wanted. The second most important instruction is to time yourself properly so that you answer every question. The third most important instruction is to answer every question. Guess if you have to but include something for each question. Remember that you will receive no credit for a blank and will probably receive some credit if you write something in answer to an essay question. If you guess a letter – say "B" for a multiple-choice question – you may have guessed right. If you leave a blank as an answer to a multiple-choice question, the examiners may respect your feelings but it will not add a point to your score. Some exams may penalize you for wrong answers, so in such cases only, you may not want to guess unless you have some basis for your answer.

7) Suggestions
   a. Objective-type questions
      1. Examine the question booklet for proper sequence of pages and questions
      2. Read all instructions carefully
      3. Skip any question which seems too difficult; return to it after all other questions have been answered
      4. Apportion your time properly; do not spend too much time on any single question or group of questions
      5. Note and underline key words – all, most, fewest, least, best, worst, same, opposite, etc.
      6. Pay particular attention to negatives
      7. Note unusual option, e.g., unduly long, short, complex, different or similar in content to the body of the question
      8. Observe the use of "hedging" words – probably, may, most likely, etc.

9. Make sure that your answer is put next to the same number as the question
10. Do not second-guess unless you have good reason to believe the second answer is definitely more correct
11. Cross out original answer if you decide another answer is more accurate; do not erase until you are ready to hand your paper in
12. Answer all questions; guess unless instructed otherwise
13. Leave time for review

b. Essay questions
1. Read each question carefully
2. Determine exactly what is wanted. Underline key words or phrases.
3. Decide on outline or paragraph answer
4. Include many different points and elements unless asked to develop any one or two points or elements
5. Show impartiality by giving pros and cons unless directed to select one side only
6. Make and write down any assumptions you find necessary to answer the questions
7. Watch your English, grammar, punctuation and choice of words
8. Time your answers; don't crowd material

8) Answering the essay question

Most essay questions can be answered by framing the specific response around several key words or ideas. Here are a few such key words or ideas:

M's: manpower, materials, methods, money, management
P's: purpose, program, policy, plan, procedure, practice, problems, pitfalls, personnel, public relations

a. Six basic steps in handling problems:
1. Preliminary plan and background development
2. Collect information, data and facts
3. Analyze and interpret information, data and facts
4. Analyze and develop solutions as well as make recommendations
5. Prepare report and sell recommendations
6. Install recommendations and follow up effectiveness

b. Pitfalls to avoid
1. Taking things for granted – A statement of the situation does not necessarily imply that each of the elements is necessarily true; for example, a complaint may be invalid and biased so that all that can be taken for granted is that a complaint has been registered
2. Considering only one side of a situation – Wherever possible, indicate several alternatives and then point out the reasons you selected the best one
3. Failing to indicate follow up – Whenever your answer indicates action on your part, make certain that you will take proper follow-up action to see how successful your recommendations, procedures or actions turn out to be
4. Taking too long in answering any single question – Remember to time your answers properly

EXAMINATION SECTION

EXAMINATION SECTION
TEST 1

DIRECTIONS: Each question or incomplete statement is followed by several suggested answers or completions. Select the one that BEST answers the question or completes the statement. *PRINT THE LETTER OF THE CORRECT ANSWER IN THE SPACE AT THE RIGHT.*

1. An indication of NO RASTER, SOUND OK is a defective
   - A. mixer oscillator
   - B. low voltage supply
   - C. CRT
   - D. video detector

2. The symptom of a HORIZONTAL LINE, SOUND OK is a defect in the
   - A. CRT
   - B. vertical sweep
   - C. horizontal sweep
   - D. video output

3. The symptom of NO RASTER, NO SOUND is caused by the
   - A. horizontal sweep
   - B. audio output
   - C. low voltage power supply
   - D. tuner

4. The symptoms of RASTER OK, NO PICTURE, NO SOUND is caused by
   - A. sound IF
   - B. 1st video IF
   - C. vertical sweep
   - D. sync

5. A tilted picture can BEST be cured by
   - A. turning the CRT
   - B. adjusting the vertical size
   - C. adjusting the yoke
   - D. moving the centering tabs

6. Failure to push the yoke against the CRT will result in
   - A. a tilted picture
   - B. ion burns
   - C. blooming
   - D. neck shadows

7. A receiver has good sound, but the screen is black. The FIRST check to make would be
   - A. replace the low voltage rectifier
   - B. draw an arc from the anode lead
   - C. adjust the brightness control
   - D. replace the CRT

8. When the picture rolls up and down, the control needing adjustment is the _____ control.
   - A. horizontal
   - B. contrast
   - C. vertical hold
   - D. sync

9. The wave shape at the grid of the horizontal amplifier is a
   - A. sinewave
   - B. sharp pulse
   - C. squarewave
   - D. sawtooth wave

10. A technician wants to observe a horizontal sync pulse on the scope. He would connect the probe to the

    A. external sweep
    B. vertical input
    C. horizontal input
    D. sync input

11. The feedback path in a cathode coupled multivibrator is supplied by

    A. a capacitor
    B. a winding from the plate to the cathode
    C. a common cathode resistor
    D. the cathode to the plate interelectrode capacitance

12. The horizontal hold control

    A. controls the vertical size
    B. controls the horizontal size
    C. varies the horizontal sweep frequency
    D. holds the horizontal oscillator up

13. The high voltage supply provides the voltage for the

    A. horizontal sweep circuit
    B. plate of the video output tube
    C. plate of the sync tube
    D. cathode ray tube

14. The high voltage is produced by the

    A. horizontal sweep signal
    B. vertical sweep signal
    C. horizontal sync pulse
    D. vertical sync pulse

15. A variable resistor in the grid of the vertical multivibrator would be called the

    A. vertical hold
    B. horizontal hold
    C. contrast control
    D. brightness control

16. The two signals that are fed to the horizontal AFC stage are the

    A. vertical and horizontal sync pulses
    B. video and horizontal sync pulses
    C. horizontal sweep signal and the horizontal sync pulse
    D. composite video and sound

17. When servicing a television, freeze spray is used to

    A. stiffen the copper wires
    B. hold printed circuit leads to the circuit board
    C. cool hot or overheated tubes
    D. locate intermittent components

18. A crosshatch generator is used by a serviceman working on a color receiver to make a(n)

    A. IF alignment
    B. dynamic convergence
    C. purity adjustment
    D. gray scale tracking

19. When colored snow (confetti) is seen on an unused channel, adjust the _____ control.   19._____

    A. AGC   B. color   C. tint   D. killer

20. A large magenta patch showing on a red screen calls for   20._____

    A. purity adjustment
    B. blue lateral adjustment
    C. horizontal dynamic convergence
    D. vertical dynamic convergence

21. Static convergence is acceptable in a color television when   21._____

    A. no color tinting shows on a black and white picture
    B. the vertical lines are converged at the top and bottom
    C. the horizontal lines are converged at the top and bottom
    D. the three beams are converged to form white dots at the center of the screen

22. What can cause ghost images on a television screen?   22._____

    A. Improper orientation of the antenna
    B. An RF amplifier with low grain
    C. A db loss in the transmission line
    D. Excessive signal strength

23. Before removing the second anode lead from the CRT, a repairman should   23._____

    A. remove the cap from the high voltage rectifier
    B. remove the high voltage rectifier
    C. short the cap of the high voltage rectifier to ground
    D. short the second anode of the CRT to the ground

24. A wide black horizontal bar across the screen on the CRT is *probably* due to   24._____

    A. 120 cycle hum,
    B. too much power supply filtering
    C. 60 cycle hum
    D. a weak rectifier tube

25. The three primary color phosphors used in color TV are   25._____

    A. red, blue, and yellow   B. red, white, and blue
    C. magenta, cyan, and yellow   D. red, green, and blue

KEY (CORRECT ANSWERS)

1. C
2. B
3. C
4. B
5. C

6. D
7. C
8. C
9. D
10. B

11. C
12. C
13. D
14. A
15. A

16. C
17. D
18. B
19. D
20. A

21. D
22. A
23. D
24. C
25. D

TEST 2

DIRECTIONS: Each question or incomplete statement is followed by several suggested answers or completions. Select the one that BEST answers the question or completes the statement. *PRINT THE LETTER OF THE CORRECT ANSWER IN THE SPACE AT THE RIGHT.*

1. A picture CANNOT be locked-in either horizontally or vertically. The fault is *probably* in the

    A. low voltage power supply
    B. sync section
    C. horizontal deflection section
    D. vertical deflection section

    1.____

2. *Barber pole* is a term commonly used to describe a lack of

    A. horizontal sync
    B. vertical blanking
    C. color sync
    D. retrace blanking

    2.____

3. The _____ amplifier is cut off by the color killer in a television receiver.

    A. band pass
    B. burst
    C. video
    D. IF

    3.____

4. Purity adjustments concern

    A. *only* statfic adjustments
    B. *only* convergence adjustments
    C. *only* yoke position adjustments
    D. yoke position and purity ring adjustments

    4.____

5. The circuit that separates the chroma signal from the composite video signal and feeds it to the demodulators is the

    A. color killer
    B. luminance amplifier
    C. bandpass amplifier
    D. burst amplifier

    5.____

6. A yellow-tinted color receiver raster indicates the absence of

    A. red   B. green   C. blue   D. yellow

    6.____

7. Automatic degaussing of MOST color television receivers occurs during the

    A. operation of the set
    B. period that the set is off
    C. initial warm-up period
    D. initial cool-off period

    7:____

8. Sound carrier interference is removed from the picture circuits by

    A. trap
    B. volume control
    C. peaking coil
    D. gate

    8.____

9. A *Keystone* pattern on the screen indicates a(n)

    A. open yoke
    B. defective damper tube
    C. shorted yoke winding
    D. open output transformer

    9.____

5

10. A defect in the sync separator stage will cause

    A. loss of raster
    B. rolling of the picture
    C. tearing of the picture
    D. rolling and tearing of the picture

11. A yoke mismatch may cause

    A. loss of contrast			B. poor AGC action
    C. loss of sync			D. ringing in the raster

12. The peak-to-peak value of the composite video signal at the output of the picture detector is _____ volts.

    A. 17.6		B. 5		C. 80		D. 117

13. Reduction of H.V. applied to the CRT anode will result in

    A. an increase in the size of the raster
    B. blooming
    C. no effect on the raster
    D. shadows on the raster

14. When aligning a video I.F. system, the important thing to look for is

    A. maximum gain
    B. picture carrier to be at exact center of the curve
    C. maximum bandwidth
    D. proper shape and bandwidth

15. Soft x-rays come from the _____ in a color TV set.

    A. vertical sweep section
    B. horizontal sweep and high voltage section
    C. sync and age section
    D. tuner

16. An inoperative oscillator stage in the tuner will result in

    A. no raster
    B. no picture and no sound
    C. no high voltage at the CRT
    D. hum bars in the picture

17. The flyback type of high voltage power supply is dependent for its operation upon the _____ output system.

    A. vertical deflection		B. AF
    C. horizontal deflection		D. video

18. Which of the following should be used to adjust the AGC level control on the keyer tube? The

    A. strongest station
    B. weakest station
    C. television set with the antenna removed
    D. lower setting on contrast

19. To fix a picture that appears to be silvery, a repairman should use a(n)

    A. isolation transformer   B. new brightness control
    C. booster   D. new video amplifier tube

20. The varactor tuner changes its oscillator frequency by varying

    A. a tuning capacitor   B. an inductor
    C. DC voltage   D. resistance

21. If the delay line opens in a color receiver, it would cause

    A. loss of color   B. a negative picture
    C. lack of color sync   D. a loss of the Y signal

22. If a cathode bias resistor in the burst amplifier circuit of a color television receiver became an open circuit, it would cause

    A. confetti
    B. a monochrome picture
    C. lack of blue hues in the picture
    D. lack of red hues in the picture

23. When adjusting the focus control of a color television receiver at normal brightness and contrast levels, the technician should observe the

    A. overall high frequency response
    B. raster or picture lines
    C. static convergence
    D. dynamic convergence

24. In a television reception area where ghosts are developed on the receiver's kine, these ghosts can be minimized by antenna orientation and by using an antenna with

    A. multiple reflectors   B. multiple directors
    C. stacked dipoles   D. folded dipoles

25. To reduce color fringes at the bottom of a monochrome picture, adjust the

    A. color level control   B. purity magnet
    C. dynamic convergence   D. color video drive signals

KEY (CORRECT ANSWERS)

1.	B	11.	D
2.	C	12.	B
3.	A	13.	B
4.	D	14.	D
5.	C	15.	B
6.	C	16.	B
7.	C	17.	C
8.	A	18.	A
9.	C	19.	C
10.	D	20.	C

21. D
22. B
23. B
24. A
25. C

EXAMINATION SECTION
TEST 1

DIRECTIONS: Each question or incomplete statement is followed by several suggested answers or completions. Select the one that BEST answers the question or completes the statement. *PRINT THE LETTER OF THE CORRECT ANSWER IN THE SPACE AT THE RIGHT.*

1. The purpose of gray scale tracking is to   1.____

    A. achieve 59% green 11% blue 30% red
    B. accomplish a pure red screen
    C. improve focus
    D. lock in picture

2. When purity is adjusted properly,   2.____

    A. color fringing is corrected
    B. a uniform red screen is accomplished
    C. the audio response is improved
    D. none of the above

3. A service switch on a color receiver is used for   3.____

    A. adjusting gray scale tracking
    B. adjusting vertical size
    C. maintaining signal levels
    D. control of synchronization

4. The function of an AFC circuit is to   4.____

    A. correct tracking automatically
    B. maintain same level for strong and weak signals
    C. control the AFC circuit
    D. none of the above

5. A yellow raster indicates the loss of   5.____

    A. R-Y   B. G-Y
    C. B-Y   D. red and green

6. An inoperative burst amplifier would cause   6.____

    A. confetti
    B. a monochrome picture
    C. no blue hues in the picture
    D. no red hues in the picture

7. When observing a horizontal sync pulse on the oscilloscope, the probe is connected to   7.____

    A. external sweep   B. sync input
    C. horizontal input   D. vertical input

9

8. To reduce color fringes at the bottom of a monochrome picture, adjust the

   A. color level control
   B. purity magnet
   C. dynamic convergence
   D. color video drive signals

9. A defect in the vertical oscillator will cause

   A. rolling
   B. picture tearing horizontally
   C. lack of contrast
   D. insufficient width

10. The wave shape at the grid of the horizontal amplifier is a

    A. sinewave
    B. sharp pulse
    C. squarewave
    D. sawtooth wave

11. The signals found at the output of the video detector are

    A. composite video
    B. audio frequency and composite video
    C. sync and sound signals
    D. composite video and 4.5 MC

12. The horizontal retrace takes place

    A. at the beginning of each line
    B. during the blanking period
    C. at the end of a field
    D. at the end of a frame

13. Special high voltage rectifier tube sockets are used to

    A. prevent high voltage arcing
    B. keep dust from the socket
    C. reduce hum
    D. avoid too much heat

14. A *balun* is used to

    A. prevent shock at the antenna
    B. reduce unwanted frequencies
    C. provide maximum signal transfer to receiver input
    D. change the directional properties of the antenna

15. The effect of a cathode to grid short in a CRT will result in

    A. ghosts
    B. a blooming picture
    C. a negative picture
    D. no control of brightness

16. The video output signal of the video detector is APPROXIMATELY _____ volts P-P.

    A. 4	B. 25	C. 40	D. 80

17. Where might soft x-rays come from in a color television set?   17.____

    A. Vertical sweep section
    B. Horizontal sweep and high voltage section
    C. Sync and AGC section
    D. Tuner

18. Reduction of H.V. applied to the CRT anode will result in   18.____

    A. an increase in the size of the raster
    B. blooming
    C. no effect on the raster
    D. shadows on the raster

19. A yoke mismatch may cause   19.____

    A. loss of contrast   B. poor AGC action
    C. loss of sync   D. ringing in the raster

20. A defect in the sync separator stage will cause   20.____

    A. loss of raster
    B. rolling of the picture
    C. tearing of the picture
    D. rolling and tearing of the picture

21. A *keystone* pattern on the screen indicates a(n)   21.____

    A. open yoke   B. defective damper tube
    C. shorted yoke winding   D. open output transformer

22. Sound carrier interference is removed from the picture circuits by a   22.____

    A. trap   B. volume control
    C. peaking coil   D. gate

23. Automatic degaussing of most color television receivers occurs during the   23.____

    A. operation of the set
    B. period that the set is off
    C. initial warm-up period
    D. initial cool-off period

24. A circuit that separates the chroma signal from the composite video signal and feeds it to   24.____
    the demodulators is the

    A. color killer   B. luminance amplifier
    C. bandpass amplifier   D. burst amplifier

25. Purity adjustments concern   25.____

    A. static adjustments *only*
    B. convergence adjustments *only*
    C. yoke position adjustments *only*
    D. yoke position and purity ring adjustments

KEY (CORRECT ANSWERS)

1.	A	11.	A
2.	A	12.	B
3.	A	13.	A
4.	C	14.	C
5.	C	15.	B
6.	B	16.	A
7.	C	17.	B
8.	B	18.	B
9.	B	19.	D
10.	D	20.	B

21. C
22. A
23. C
24. B
25. A

———

TEST 2

DIRECTIONS: Each question or incomplete statement is followed by several suggested answers or completions. Select the one that BEST answers the question or completes the statement. *PRINT THE LETTER OF THE CORRECT ANSWER IN THE SPACE AT THE RIGHT.*

1. When adjusting the focus control of a color television receiver at normal brightness and contrast levels, the technician should observe the

    A. overall high frequency response
    B. raster or picture lines
    C. static convergence
    D. dynamic convergence

    1.____

2. A Crosshatch generator is used by a serviceman working on a color receiver to make a(n)

    A. IF alignment
    B. dynamic convergence
    C. purity adjustment
    D. gray scale tracking

    2.____

3. A variable resistor in the grid of the vertical multivibrator is called the

    A. vertical hold
    B. horizontal hold
    C. contrast control
    D. brightness control

    3.____

4. An inoperative oscillator stage in the tuner will result in

    A. no raster
    B. no picture and no sound
    C. no high voltage at the CRT
    D. hum bars in the picture

    4.____

5. The high voltage is produced by the

    A. horizontal sweep signal
    B. vertical sweep signal
    C. horizontal sync pulse
    D. none of the above

    5.____

6. The flyback type of high voltage power supply is dependent for its operation upon the _____ system.

    A. vertical deflection output
    B. AF output
    C. horizontal deflection output
    D. video output

    6.____

7. The varactor tuner changes its oscillator frequency by varying

    A. a tuning capacitor
    B. an inductor
    C. the DC voltage
    D. the resistance

    7.____

8. The feedback path in an emitter coupled multivibrator is supplied by

    A. a capacitor
    B. a winding from the plate to the cathode
    C. a common emitter resistor
    D. the cathode to the plate interelectrode capacitance

    8.____

9. A picture cannot be locked in either horizontally or vertically. The fault is PROBABLY in the

   A. low voltage power supply
   B. sync section
   C. horizontal deflection section
   D. vertical deflection section

10. The three primary color phosphors used in color TV are

    A. red, blue, and yellow
    B. red, white, and blue
    C. magenta, cyan, and yellow
    D. red, green, and blue

11. Before removing the second anode lead from the CRT, a repairman should

    A. remove the cap from the high voltage rectifier
    B. remove the high voltage rectifier
    C. short the cap of the high voltage
    D. short the second anode of the CRT to the ground

12. A large magenta patch showing on a red screen calls for

    A. purity adjustment
    B. blue lateral adjustment
    C. horizontal dynamic convergence
    D. vertical dynamic convergence

13. What can cause ghost images on a television screen?

    A. Improper orientation of the antenna
    B. An RF amplifier with low grain
    C. A db loss in the transmission line
    D. Excessive signal strength

14. Static convergence is acceptable in a color television when

    A. no color tinting shows on a black and white picture
    B. the vertical lines are converged at the top and bottom
    C. the horizontal lines are converged at the top and bottom
    D. the three beams are converged to form white dots at the center of the screen

15. When colored snow (confetti) is seen on an unused channel, adjust the _____ control.

    A. AGC   B. color   C. tint   D. killer

16. A receiver has good sound but the screen is black. The FIRST check to make would be

    A. replace the low voltage rectifier
    B. draw an arc from the anode lead
    C. adjust the brightness control
    D. replace the CRT

17. The horizontal hold controls the

    A. vertical size (height)
    B. horizontal size (width)
    C. horizontal oscillator up
    D. none of the above

18. The symptom of raster ok, no picture, no sound is caused by

    A. sound IF   B. 1st video IF
    C. vertical sweep   D. sync

19. An indication of no raster, sound ok is a defective

    A. mixer oscillator   B. low voltage supply
    C. CRT   D. video detector

20. Which amplifier is cut off by the color killer in a television receiver?

    A. Band pass   B. Burst
    C. Video   D. IF

KEY (CORRECT ANSWERS)

1.	D	11.	C
2.	B	12.	A
3.	A	13.	A
4.	B	14.	A
5.	C	15.	D
6.	C	16.	C
7.	C	17.	B
8.	A	18.	B
9.	B	19.	C
10.	D	20.	B

EXAMINATION SECTION
TEST 1

DIRECTIONS: Each question or incomplete statement is followed by several suggested answers or completions. Select the one that BEST answers the question or completes the statement. *PRINT THE LETTER OF THE CORRECT ANSWER IN THE SPACE AT THE RIGHT.*

1. The length of a Marconi-type antenna is _____ wavelength.
   A. ¼   B. ½   C. ¾   D. 1

2. A whip antenna of less than ¼ wavelength will present an electrical impedance that is
   A. resistive
   B. capacitive
   C. inductive
   D. 180° out-of-phase

3. Frequency multiplication is achieved in transmitter stages by operating them as Class _____ amplifiers.
   A. A   B. AB   C. B   D. C

4. The power factor of a resonant circuit is
   A. lagging   B. leading   C. unity   D. zero

5. The power factor of a *parallel* circuit consisting of a 51-ohm resistor and a 51-ohm capacitive reactance is
   A. .500   B. .667   C. .707   D. .887

6. A tunable *series* RLC circuit will have MINIMUM impedance when the
   A. capacitive reactance equals the inductive reactance
   B. inductive reactance or capacitive reactance equals zero
   C. capacitive reactance equals the resistance
   D. inductive reactance equals the resistance

7. At resonance, a tunable *parallel* RLC circuit will be characterized by
   A. broadest bandwidth
   B. lowest "Q"
   C. maximum impedance
   D. equal currents through the resistance, inductance, and capacitance

8. If the number of turns of an inductor is halved, the value of the inductance is
   A. doubled
   B. unchanged
   C. reduced to one-half
   D. reduced to one-quarter

9. The resistivity of copper is GREATER than that of the element
   A. silicon   B. germanium   C. silver   D. gold

10. The MINIMUM number of 10-microfarad, 25-volt capacitors that can be connected up to yield an equivalent capacitance of 5 microfarads, usable on 150 volts, is
    A. 2   B. 6   C. 18   D. 24

11. The number of DB's (decibels) corresponding to a power ratio of 200 is MOST NEARLY _____ DB's.
    A. 20   B. 23   C. 26   D. 40

12. The MAXIMUM current carrying capacity, in amperes, of a resistor marked "5,000 ohms, 200 watts" is
    A. 1/25   B. 1/5   C. 5   D. 25

13. The combined equivalent resistance of a 12-ohm resistor, a 6-ohm resistor, and a 4-ohm resistor connected in *parallel* is
    A. ½ ohm   B. 1 ohm   C. 2 ohms   D. 3 ohms

14. The percentage regulation of a power supply with a no-load voltage output of +25.3 volts and a full-load voltage output of +23.0 volts is
    A. 1.9%   B. 2.1%   C. 9%   D. 10%

15. A capacitance of .0015 microfarads is equal to
    A. 150 picofarads
    B. 1500 picofarads
    C. 150 nanofarads
    D. 1500 nanofarads

16. A diode is color coded with a purple, a green, and a red ring in that order (the purple ring is at the end of the diode). It should be concluded from the coding that the diode is a
    A. IN752   B. IN7500   C. IN75B   D. IN7511

17. The time constant of a resistance and an inductance in *series* can be increased by
    A. *increasing* either the resistance or the inductance
    B. *increasing* the resistance or decreasing the inductance
    C. *decreasing* the resistance or increasing the inductance
    D. *decreasing* either the resistance or the inductance

18. The combined equivalent impedance of a 50-ohm inductive reactance connected in *parallel* with a 25-ohm capacitive reactance is
    A. 75 ohms inductive reactance
    B. 75 ohms capacitive reactance
    C. 50 ohms inductive reactance
    D. 50 ohms capacitive reactance

19. The tree connections of an SCR are the
    A. collector, emitter, and gate
    B. base 1, base 2, and emitter
    C. anode, cathode, and gate
    D. emitter 1, emitter 2, and base

20. FET is the abbreviation for a _____ transistor.
    A. fast epitaxial
    B. field effect
    C. frequency extended
    D. forward emitting

3 (#1)

21. The resonant frequency of a .1 henry inductance and a .001 microfarad capacitance "tank" circuit is MOST NEARLY
    A. 160 Hz   B. 1600 Hz   C. 16 KHz   D. 16 MHz

22. At 300 MHz, electromagnetic energy in air has a wavelength of
    A. 1 centimeter   B. 10 centimeters
    C. 100 centimeters   D. 1000 centimeters

23. The frequency range from 300 MHz to 3000 MHz is designated by RETMA and ASA as the _____ range.
    A. HF   B. VHF   C. UHF   D. SHF

24. A modulated carrier wave has a maximum magnitude of 150 volts and 50% modulation.
    If the modulation is removed, the carrier will have a magnitude of _____ volts.
    A. 50   B. 75   C. 100   D. 150

25. If 50 microamperes produces a full-scale deflection on a DC voltmeter, the sensitivity of the instrument is _____ ohms/volt.
    A. 5,000   B. 10,000   C. 20,000   D. 50,000

26. A "beat-frequency meter" is also called a
    A. frequency synthesizer   B. distortion meter
    C. wave analyzer   D. heterodyne-frequency meter

27. Assume that a voltmeter uses the same scale for three ranges, 0-300 volts, 0-75 volts, and 0-15 volts.
    If the scale is marked only for the 0-300 volt range, then a scale reading of 120 when the 0-75 volt range is being used will correspond to an ACTUAL voltage of _____ volts.
    A. 10   B. 12   C. 24   D. 30

28. Variations in the signals introduced in the "Z" axis input of an oscilloscope produce corresponding changes in the
    A. positioning of the time-delayed sweep
    B. intensity of the trace
    C. "Y" axis frequency response
    D. "X" axis sawtooth repetition rate

29. When using an ohmmeter to measure resistance, the GREATEST accuracy is obtained when the range selected results in a deflection that is APPROXIMATELY
    A. ¼ full-scale   B. ½ full-scale
    C. ¾ full-scale   D. full-scale

30. A grid-dip meter is GENERALLY used to measure
    A. Q   B. modulation   C. RF current   D. frequency

31. A 0-150 volt voltmeter has an accuracy of 2% F.S.
When the pointer shows 75 volts, the MAXIMUM error is plus or minus
   A. .5 volt   B. 1.5 volts   C. 2.0 volts   D. 3.0 volts

32. Certain attenuation probes used with oscilloscopes provide for an adjustment to be made in each probe, prior to its use. The adjustment is required in order to _____ on which it is used.
   A. match the probe to the circuitry
   B. match the probe to the input of the scope
   C. adjust the DC volts/division sensitivity of the input to the scope
   D. adjust the DC balance of the input to the scope

33. When an oscilloscope is set up to display a lissajous pattern, the feature that is inhibited and NOT available is the
   A. "Y" axis manual positioning control
   B. "X" axis manual positioning control
   C. automatic retrace blanking
   D. trace intensity manual control

34. In order to minimize multiple reflections in a coaxial line, the MOST effective steps that should be taken are to drive the sending end with a
   A. low impedance source and terminate the receiving end with a resistance equal to the coaxial characteristic impedance
   B. source with output impedance equal to the coaxial characteristic impedance and terminate the receiving end with a resistance equal to the coaxial characteristic impedance
   C. low impedance source and terminate the receiving end with a high impedance
   D. source with output impedance to the coaxial characteristic impedance and terminate the receiving end with a high impedance

35. Of the following statements concerning a dual-trace oscilloscope, the one which is CORRECT is that it
   A. requires a two-gun cathode-ray tube
   B. has two "Y" axis inputs that are chopped and displayed as a single trace
   C. uses a single time base when used in the "chopped" mode
   D. uses dual-time bases when used in the "chopped" mode

36. The type of display usually produced on oscilloscopes, where signal amplitude is convert4ed to a "Y" axis displacement and a time base is introduced on the "X" axis, is CLOSEST in appearance to the radar indicator that is called a(n) _____ scan.
   A. A   B. B   C. J   D. PPI

37. Of the following, the BEST instrument for measuring very low resistances is the _____ bridge.
   A. Wien   B. Kelvin   C. Hay   D. Maxwell

38. Of the following, the instrument that should be used in measuring radiation patterns produced by antennas is the
    A. spectrum analyzer
    B. field-strength meter
    C. curve tracer
    D. distortion meter

38.____

39. Taut-band suspension is a feature which is incorporated in
    A. the internal supporting of hermetic-sealed units
    B. low-friction meter movements
    C. dial cord assemblies
    D. vibration mounts for electronic packages

39.____

40. A "bolometer" is a device that can be used for measuring
    A. microwave power
    B. static charge
    C. magnetic-field strength
    D. vibration frequencies

40.____

KEY (CORRECT ANSWERS)

1.	A	11.	B	21.	C	31.	D
2.	B	12.	B	22.	C	32.	B
3.	D	13.	C	23.	C	33.	C
4.	C	14.	D	24.	C	34.	B
5.	C	15.	B	25.	C	35.	C
6.	A	16.	A	26.	D	36.	A
7.	C	17.	C	27.	D	37.	B
8.	D	18.	D	28.	B	38.	B
9.	C	19.	C	29.	B	39.	B
10.	C	20.	B	30.	D	40.	A

TEST 2

DIRECTIONS: Each question or incomplete statement is followed by several suggested answers or completions. Select the one that BEST answers the question or completes the statement. *PRINT THE LETTER OF THE CORRECT ANSWER IN THE SPACE AT THE RIGHT.*

1. One of the reasons why radiotelephones are operated in the 30 MHz to 3000 MHz range is that
     A. skip transmission is very effective
     B. antenna orientation is not important
     C. the number of voice channels is great
     D. AM operation is less noisy than FM

    1.____

2. The transmission of a distress message by a radiotelephone station not itself in distress should include calling out three times the expression
     A. SOS   B. SOS relay   C. Mayday   D. Mayday relay

    2.____

3. In specifying the characteristics of an oscillator crystal, the information that should be given, together with the frequency tolerance, is the crystal
     A. age   B. operating temperature range
     C. manufacturer   D. power supply voltages

    3.____

4. Records indicate that a component in a certain unit has been replaced repeatedly, and no such history exists in other similar units with the same type of service and total operation time.
   Based on this information, it should be concluded that
     A. the replacement components were defective
     B. the component was replaced at times when it had not failed
     C. the replacement components were connected into the circuit improperly
     D. there is something else wrong in the unit causing the component to fail

    4.____

5. When trouble-shooting a large electronic unit, such as a console, first, power should be removed and the NEXT step should be that
     A. internal capacitors be discharged by using a shorting connection to chassis
     B. ohmmeter checks be made according to the instruction manual
     C. the operating personnel be notified that the unit is out of operation
     D. the door and panel interlocks be by-passed

    5.____

6. Metal enclosures and panels of electronic or electrical equipment should be well grounded in order to
     A. protect operating personnel from getting electric shocks
     B. insure that the contained equipment has a good reference ground
     C. prevent static charges from building up on the frame
     D. provide a solid mounting for the equipment and keep it firmly in place

    6.____

7. The main reason for NOT using carbon tetrachloride as a cleaning agent on electrical equipment is that it
   A. is an electrical conductor
   B. is too expensive
   C. generates toxic fumes
   D. coats equipment with an acid deposit

   7.____

8. The MOST likely cause of damage occurring in transistorized circuitry during the process of soldering is due to the application of too much
   A. pressure   B. heat   C. solder   D. rosin flux

   8.____

9. A 2-inch diameter hole can be made quickly and cleanly in a 16-gauge aluminum plate by the use of a
   A. rat-tail file   B. nibbler
   C. chassis punch   D. jig saw

   9.____

10. A reason for using teflon insulation rather than vinyl on electrical wiring is that teflon is
    A. better for bonding   B. more flexible
    C. less expensive   D. more resistant to heat

    10.____

11. Of the following statements concerning epoxy glue, the one which is CORRECT is that it
    A. dissolves quickly upon contact with water
    B. is prepared from two components that are mixed together shortly before use
    C. is a long-time favorite for making temporary bonds
    D. generally does not require clamps, nails or presses on surfaces to be joined

    11.____

12. Of the following chemicals, the one which will burn on contact with a lighted match is
    A. carbon tetrachloride   B. acetone
    C. methylene chloride   D. sodium bicarbonate

    12.____

13. Of the following, the BEST method of disposing of spray cans that contain aerosol paints or solvents is
    A. puncturing the cans and then throwing them into an incinerator
    B. puncturing the cans and then having them picked up by the sanitation men
    C. throwing them into an incinerator
    D. having them picked up by the sanitation men

    13.____

14. An ohmmeter of known polarity is connected from the base to the emitter on a transistor in such manner that the positive lead is on the base. The ohmmeter registers continuity with such conditions and then registers an "open" circuit when the leads are reversed.
    Based on this information, it should be concluded that the transistor is
    A. good   B. defective   C. an NPN   D. a PNP

    14.____

15. An ohmmeter registers "open" when connected from the emitter to the collector of a transistor (base left disconnected) and also registers "open" when the leads are reversed. This information suggests that the transistor is
    A. possibly good
    B. definitely defective
    C. an NPN
    D. a PNP

15._____

16. In order to get good indications when checking a transistor by using an ohmmeter, yet not cause damage, the voltage across the test leads should _____ 1.5 volts DC and the ohmmeter scale _____ be less than R × 100.
    A. *exceed*; should
    B. *exceed*; should not
    C. *not exceed*; should
    D. *not* exceed; should not

16._____

17. If an audio amplifier requiring a 3200-ohm load is connected to the primary winding of a 20:1 step-down output transformer, the matching speaker to be connected to the secondary winding should have an impedance of _____ ohms.
    A. 4
    B. 8
    C. 16
    D. 32

17._____

18. The converter stage in a typical heterodyne receiver combines the functions of a(n)
    A. RF stage and the local oscillator
    B. mixer stage and the local oscillator
    C. RF stage and an IF stage
    D. mixer stage and an IF stage

18._____

19. One of the reasons why RF stages improve the performance of a typical heterodyne receiver is that they
    A. increase the sensitivity and broaden the bandwidth
    B. provide regenerative action and improve selectivity
    C. increase sensitivity and improve AVC action
    D. improve AVC action and broaden bandwidth

19._____

20. Of the following statements concerning the record heads in typical magnetic-tape recorders, the one which is CORRECT is that they are
    A. self-cleaning and require occasional realignment
    B. automatically demagnetized by the signals in the tape-erase heads
    C. easily magnetized and should not be checked for continuity with an ohmmeter
    D. not self-cleaning and are demagnetized by over-driving the record amplifiers

20._____

21. Typical recording speeds on commercial magnetic-tape recorders are
    A. 3½ ips, 7 ips, 15 ips, and 30 ips
    B. 3¾ ips, 7 ½ ips, 15 ips, and 30 ips
    C. 3¾ ips, 7 ips, 15 ips, and 25 ips
    D. 3½ ips, 7½ ips, 15 ips, and 30 ips

21._____

22. According to FCC regulations, the frequency and deviation of a crystal-controlled FM transmitter must be checked BEFORE it is put into operation, and rechecked thereafter every
    A. month   B. 3 months   C. 6 months   D. year

23. According to FCC regulations, radio transmitters may be tuned or adjusted only by persons possessing a
    A. first or second class commercial radiotelephone operator's license
    B. first class commercial radiotelephone operator's license
    C. first or second class commercial radiotelephone operator's license or by personnel working under their immediate supervision
    D. first class commercial radiotelephone operator's license or by personnel working under their immediate supervision

24. According to FCC regulations, transmitters whose oscillators are not crystal controlled should have their carrier frequencies checked BEFORE they are put into operation, and rechecked thereafter every
    A. week   B. month   C. 3 months   D. 6 months

25. The FCC dictates that the power in the output stage(s) of a 5-watt transmitter, whose modulation and power setting remain unaltered, should be checked at the time it is put into operation, and rechecked thereafter every
    A. month   B. 3 months   C. 6 months   D. year

Questions 26-40.

DIRECTIONS: Questions 26 through 40 are to be answered on the basis of the schematic diagram appearing on pages 7 (#2) and 8 (#2).

26. The circuits shown on the schematic represent the stages of a(n)
    A. transmitter   B. receiver
    C. audio-intercom   D. pulse-generator

27. The types of transistors shown on the schematic are
    A. all NPN's
    B. all PNP's
    C. some NPN's and some PNP's
    D. interchangeable and usable as either NPN's or PNP's

28. The power supply shown on the schematic supplies the stages with
    A. one B+ voltage, common to all stages
    B. two B+ voltages
    C. one B+ voltage and one B- voltage
    D. two B- voltages

29. The circuit element designated as Y101, in Oscillator F1 is a
    A. remote-bias adjustment   B. compensated-crystal assembly
    C. solid-stage switching device D. protective interlock

30. If the unmodulated frequency at the collector of Q107, of the Final Amplifier, is 135 MHz, then the input frequency to the base of transistor Q103, in the Modulator is _____ MHz.
    A. 3.75　　　　B. 7.50　　　　C. 15.0　　　　D. 22.5

31. The component in the Automatic Drive Limiter that has the designation RT101,10K is a
    A. high-resistance incandescent lamp
    B. thermistor
    C. precision wire-wound resistor
    D. ballast lamp

32. The component in the power supply that has the designation of CR103 is a
    A. double-anode clipper　　　　B. tunnel diode
    C. zener diode　　　　　　　　D. rectifier bridge

33. The transistor-stage configuration in which transistor 0109 of the Integrator is connected is called a(n) _____ connection.
    A. emitter-follower　　　　B. phase-splitter
    C. Darlington　　　　　　　D. common-base

34. The component between the Amplifier-Clipper and the Integrator that has the designation L116,0.8H is a(n)
    A. air-core choke　　　　B. iron-core inductor
    C. ferrite inductor　　　　D. saturable-core inductor

35. Trouble has developed in a unit whose schematic is the one accompanying this test. DC measurements are taken and indicate that the voltage on the base of Q109 in the Integrator stage has gone to -5.6 volts and the emitter voltage has gone to 0.0 volts.
    Of the following, the condition that causes such voltage levels is
    A. the R128 potentiometer slider-arm is making poor contact
    B. Q109 has developed an "open" between base and emitter
    C. C153 has become shorted
    D. Q108, in the previous stage, has gone to cut-off

36. If, in the Pre-Amplifier stage shown in the schematic pacitor C164 were to short, the result would be that
    A. Q110 would go harder into conduction
    B. Q110 would approach cut-off
    C. Q110 would become damaged
    D. C165 would break down in the reverse direction

37. In the power supply section, capacitor C156 is required in shunt with C155 because
    A. the circuit requires a capacity of slightly more than 15 microfarads; hence, C256 would supply the additional amount
    B. C155 regulates the DC voltage while C156 shunts out ripple frequencies

C. C155 is effective in filtering low frequencies, and C156 is effective in filtering high frequencies
D. C155 and C156, in parallel, form a "pi" section of the filter network

38. R113 and C124 in the collector circuit of Q104 in the second Tripler stage form what is COMMONLY called a _____ network.
    A. self-bias
    B. low-frequency peaking
    C. parasitic-suppressor
    D. decoupling

38.____

39. The Z101 sub-miniature harmonic filter, at the output of the Final Amplifier, is a _____ filter
    A. lo-pass
    B. hi-pass
    C. notch
    D. bandpass

39.____

40. The purpose of C101, in Oscillator F1, is to
    A. adjust the bias level of the stage
    B. slightly "pull" the frequency of oscillation
    C. tune out the inductance seen looking into the transistor base
    D. suppress parasitic oscillations

40.____

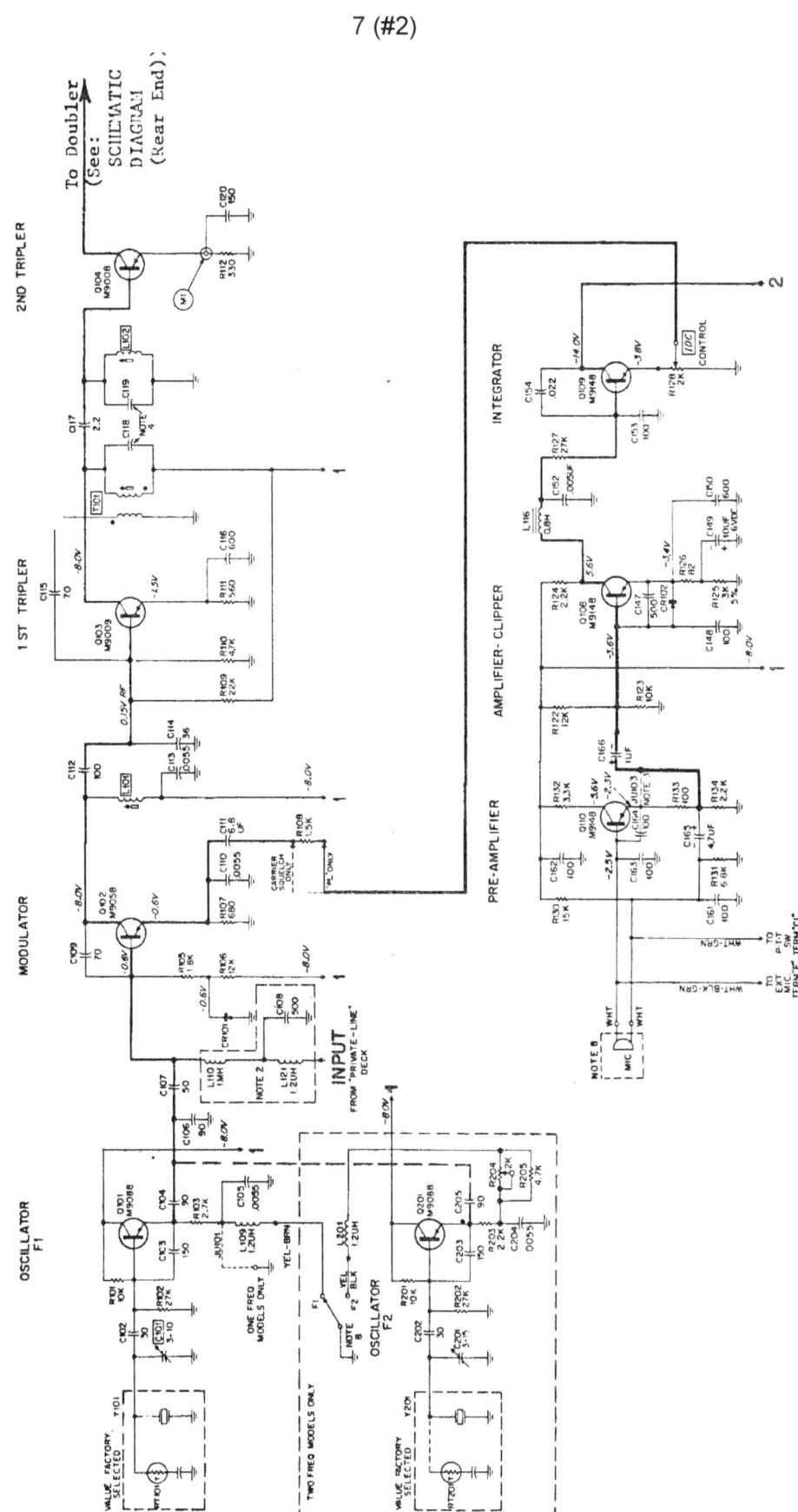

SCHEMATIC DIAGRAM (Front End)

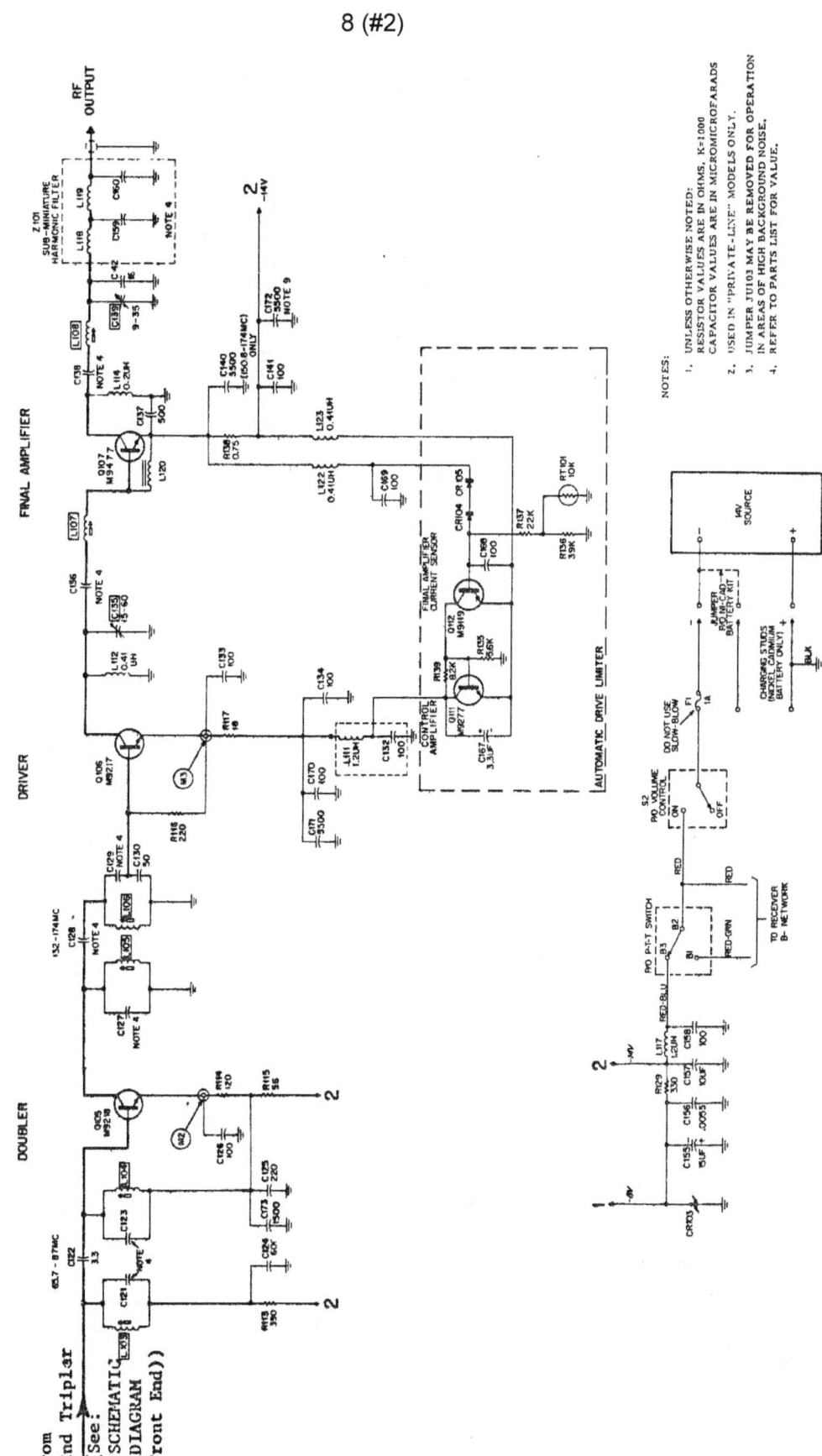

SCHEMATIC DIAGRAM (Rear End)

KEY (CORRECT ANSWERS)

1.	C	11.	B	21.	B	31.	B
2.	D	12.	B	22.	D	32.	C
3.	B	13.	D	23.	C	33.	A
4.	D	14.	C	24.	B	34.	B
5.	A	15.	A	25.	D	35.	B
6.	A	16.	D	26.	A	36.	B
7.	C	17.	B	27.	C	37.	C
8.	B	18.	B	28.	D	38.	D
9.	C	19.	C	29.	B	39.	A
10.	D	20.	C	30.	B	40.	B

TEST 3

DIRECTIONS: Each question or incomplete statement is followed by several suggested answers or completions. Select the one that BEST answers the question or completes the statement. *PRINT THE LETTER OF THE CORRECT ANSWER IN THE SPACE AT THE RIGHT.*

1. If an amplifier has three stages each having a gain of ten, the overall gain of the amplifier is
   A. 30   B. 300   C. 1,000   D. 1,000,000

   1._____

2. An amplitude-modulated carrier is said to be overmodulated when the
   A. carrier amplitude sometimes is zero for an appreciable time
   B. audio frequencies exceed the assigned bandwidth
   C. audio frequencies are close to the carrier frequency
   D. carrier amplitude sometimes exceeds the rated tank voltage

   2._____

3. For a radio receiver in which the tuning is done with variable air condensers, the practical ratio of highest to lowest frequency that can be tuned with a single coil for each condenser is NEAREST to
   A. 1.5:1   B. 3:1   C. 6:1   D. 12:1

   3._____

4. A 2k-ohm, a 4k-ohm, a 6k-ohm, and an 8k-ohm resistor are connected in parallel to a 100-volt power source. The resistor which must have the HIGHEST rating, in watts, is the
   A. 2k-ohm   B. 4k-ohm   C. 6k-ohm   D. 8k-ohm

   4._____

5. A large number of 10-microfarad, 25-volt condensers are available in a particular laboratory. The MINIMUM number of these required to yield a capacitance of 5 microfarads for operation on 150 volts is
   A. 2   B. 6   C. 18   D. 24

   5._____

6. The heaters of three vacuum tubes are to be operated in series with a resistor on a 120-volt circuit.
   If the ratings of the heaters are respectively 50, 35, and 12 volts, all at 0.15 amp, the MINIMUM rating of the resistor should be
   A. 250 ohms; 5 watts   B. 250 ohms, 10 watts
   C. 150 ohms, 10 watts   D. 150 ohms, 5 watts

   6._____

7. An audio amplifier is stated to have a frequency response of ±3 db from 50 to 10,000 cps. If the response is down 3 db at 50 cycles, the voltage output at this frequency (50 cycles) compared to the average voltage output throughout the frequency range is ABOUT
   A. 50%   B. 63%   C. 67%   d. 70%

   7._____

8. The MAXIMUM limits of resistance of a resistor having yellow, green, and orange color bands (reading from left to right) are
   A. 44,100 – 45,900   B. 42,750 – 47,250
   C. 41,500 – 49,500   D. 36,000 – 54,000

   8._____

2 (#3)

9. A COMMONLY used IF for FM receivers in the 88-108 mc. range is
   A. 455 kc.   B. 456 kc.   C. 10.7 mc.   D. 22.3 mc.

9._____

10. Crystal controlled oscillator frequency stability is maintained MOST closely by
    A. feeding the output into a tuned tank circuit
    B. enclosing the crystal in a temperature controlled oven
    C. mounting the crystal in a shock-proof container
    D. obtaining the input from a tuned tank circuit

10._____

11. One COMMONLY used dual triode vacuum tube has the designation
    A. 12AU7   B. 12BE6   C. 12SA7   D. 12SQ7

11._____

12. The base radiotelephone station used for contacting surface line patrol cars in operation 24 hours per day would be meeting legal requirements if self-identification were made
    A. 24 times a day   B. every 2 hours
    C. at the end of each transmission   D. at the beginning of each day

12._____

13. The alphabet used in radiotelephone communication is
    A. Morse   B. international
    C. telephonic   D. phonetic

13._____

14. A d.c. meter which gives full-scale deflection at 50 microamperes has a sensitivity of _____ ohms/volt.
    A. 1,000   B. 5,000   C. 20,000   D. 50,000

14._____

15. A certain d.c. meter which gives full-scale deflection at 50 microamperes has a resistance of 250 ohms. When used to measure current, it reads .50 of full-scale with a 2.5-ohm resistor connected across the meter terminals. The measured current, in milliamperes, is NEAREST to
    A. 1.3   B. 2.5   C. 12.5   D. 25.3

15._____

16. A certain train to wayside communication system operates at a frequency of 180 mc. This corresponds to a wavelength of
    A. 1667 meters   B. 166.7 meters
    C. 1667 centimeters   D. 166.7 centimeters

16._____

17. In an FM receiver using vacuum tubes, the tube having the lowest voltage applied to the plate is USUALLY the
    A. mixer   B. IF amplifier   C. limiter   D. AF amplifier

17._____

18. A grid-dip meter is GENERALLY used to measure
    A. frequency   B. RF current   C. AF current   D. modulation

18._____

19. To obtain a trapezoidal modulation pattern on the oscilloscope, the signal applied to the horizontal deflection plates should be a
    A. square wave
    B. saw-tooth wave
    C. sample of the final tank-circuit voltage
    D. sample of the audio modulating voltage

20. To obtain a wave-envelope modulation pattern on the oscilloscope, the signal applied to the horizontal deflection plates should be a
    A. square wave
    B. saw-tooth wave
    C. sample of the audio modulating voltage
    D. sample of the final tank-circuit voltage

21. When soldering transistorized circuitry, the transistors are MOST likely to be damaged from the use of too much
    A. solder   B. rosin flux   C. heat   D. pressure

Questions 22-28.

DIRECTIONS: Questions 22 through 28 are to be answered on the basis of the following circuit.

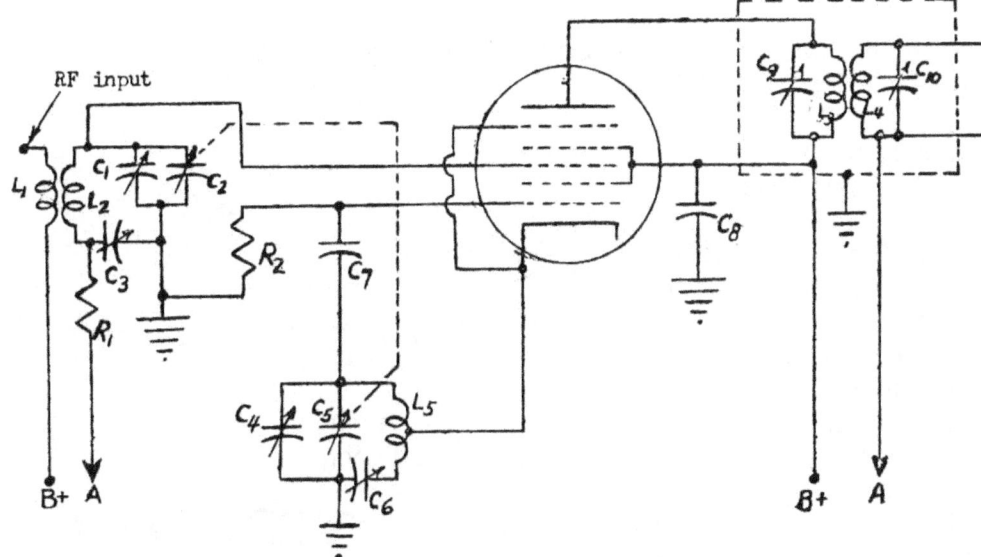

22. The name MOST commonly given to this circuit is
    A. radio-frequency amplifier   B. first detector
    C. intermediate frequency amplifier   D. ratio detector

23. The vacuum tube shown is a
    A. power amplifier pentode   B. beam power pentode
    C. hexode mixer   D. pentagrid converter

24. The wires terminating in arrowheads and labeled A MOST likely connect to the
    A. chassis
    B. AVC bus
    C. cathode bias resistors
    D. power supply screen grid bias

    24.____

25. Tracking at the high-frequency end of the tuning range is synchronized by adjusting
    A. C_1 and C_4 B. C_3 and C_6 C. C_2 and C_5 D. C_3 and C_4

    25.____

26. Tracking at the low-frequency end of the tuning range is synchronized by adjusting
    A. C_1 and C_4 B. C_3 and C_6 C. C_2 and C_5 D. C_3 and C_4

    26.____

27. The circuit shows that there is shielding around the
    A. RF tuning stage
    B. oscillator
    C. vacuum tube
    D. IF transformer

    27.____

28. The type of oscillator shown is a
    A. tickler   B. Colpitts   C. Hartley   D. TPTG

    28.____

29. A 35-ohm, 2-watt, 10% tolerance resistor should have color bands, reading from left to right, of
    A. orange, green, brown, silver
    B. orange, green, brown, gold
    C. orange, green, black, silver
    D. orange, green, black, gold

    29.____

30. The resistor of Question 29 above has a current-carrying capacity of
    A. .239 ma   B. 2.39 ma   C. 23.9 ma   D. 239 ma

    30.____

31. The 20,000 ohms/volt meter having a full-scale deflection of 50 volts reads 45 volts with switch S closed in position 1, and 21 volts when the switch is in position 2 as shown. The value of R is readily calculated to be
    A. .875 megohm
    B. 1.14 megohms
    C. 87,500 ohm
    D. 114,000 ohms

    31.____

32. In the high rejection-ratio trap circuit shown, the device that must be connected between terminals 1 and 2 for proper rejection is a(n)
    A. resistor
    B. RF choke
    C. AF choke
    D. capacitor

    32.____

33. A band elimination filter is MOST accurately illustrated by 33.____

34. The circuit which can yield a relatively sharp pulse output to the grid and cathode of a vacuum tube when a square wave is applied to the input is 34.____

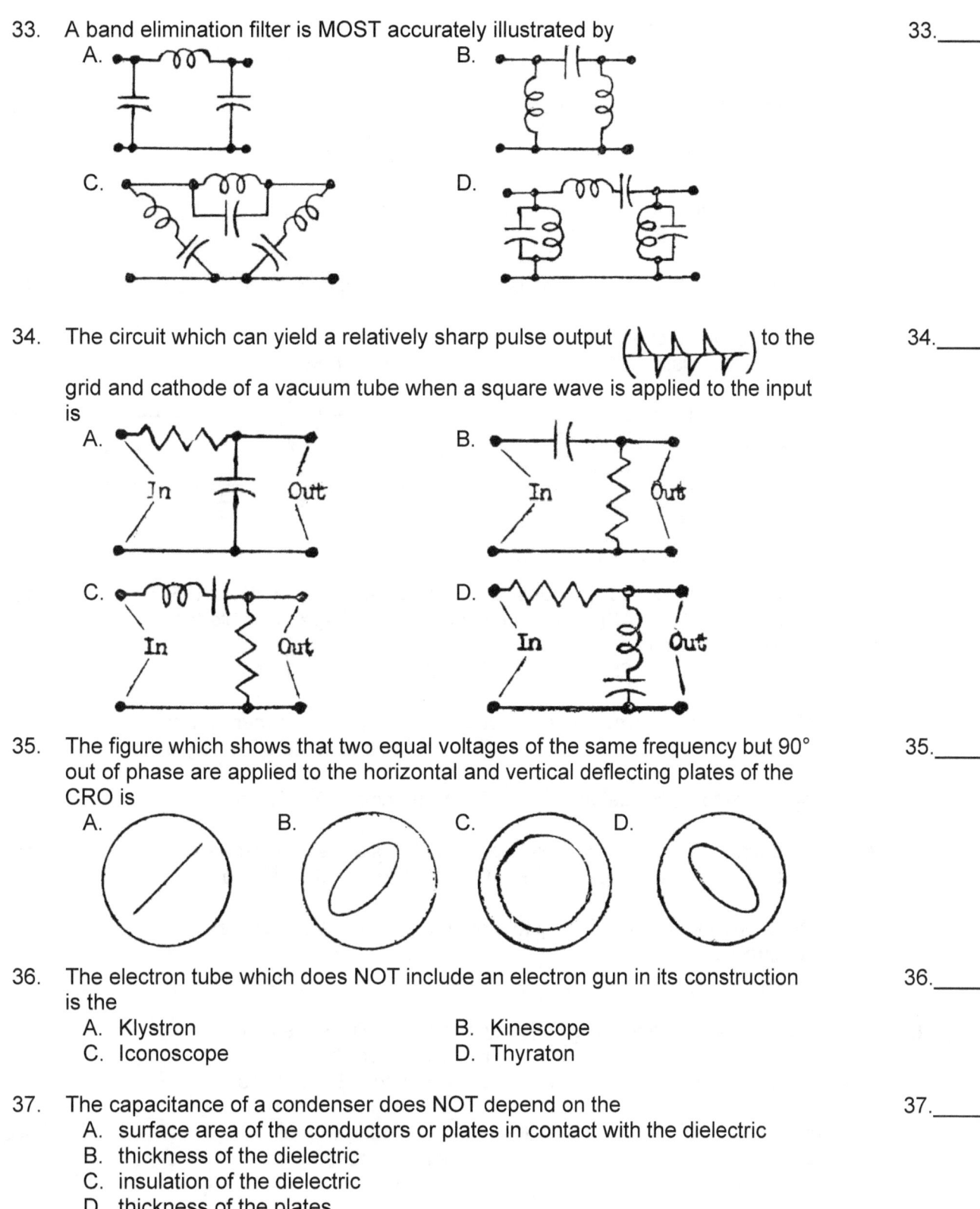

35. The figure which shows that two equal voltages of the same frequency but 90° out of phase are applied to the horizontal and vertical deflecting plates of the CRO is 35.____

36. The electron tube which does NOT include an electron gun in its construction is the 36.____
    A. Klystron
    B. Kinescope
    C. Iconoscope
    D. Thyraton

37. The capacitance of a condenser does NOT depend on the 37.____
    A. surface area of the conductors or plates in contact with the dielectric
    B. thickness of the dielectric
    C. insulation of the dielectric
    D. thickness of the plates

38. Frequency doublers and triplers are used in _____ transmitters.
    A. CW   B. pulsed   C. FM   D. keyed

39. Zener diodes are GENERALLY used for
    A. AVC rectification   B. diode detection
    C. voltage regulation   D. current limitation

40. An AF amplifier transistor could have the designation
    A. 2N243   B. 242N2   C. 1N105   D. 105N1

41. Carrier frequency voice transmission is used in wire telephony PRIMARILY to increase the
    A. number of voice channels   B. clarity of tone
    C. transmission distance   D. transmitted power

42. The circuit shown at the right is PROPERLY called a
    A. potentiometer
    B. voltage divider
    C. voltage decade
    D. current limiter

43. If R_1, R_2, and R_3 in the sketch of Question 42 above are 250k, 500k, and 50k ohms, respectively, the MAXIUM grid bias (negative) voltage available for a tube with a grounded cathode is
    A. 12.5   B. 25   C. 125   D. 250

44. Automobiles now use alternators and rectifiers instead of d.c. generators for supplying the cars' electrical demands. The rectifier that is MOST widely used is the
    A. copper oxide   B. galena   C. germanium   D. silicon

45. A circuit configuration which does NOT apply to transistors is common
    A. emitter   B. base   C. cathode   D. collector

46. The microphone that is MOST likely to require a preamplifier to operate an audio amplifier is the
    A. crystal   B. carbon   C. ceramic   D. magnetic

47. If the oscillator of a tape recorder is faulty, the MOST likely result will be
    A. incomplete erasure   B. weak recording
    C. excessive volume   D. variation in tape speed

48. Measurement of radiation from a radio antenna is made with a
    A. Q meter   B. field strength meter
    C. flux meter   D. radiometer

49. If a 0-150 volt meter is guaranteed to have an accuracy of 2% of full-scale deflection, then the MAXIMUM error of the indication when the pointer shows 25 volts is plus or minus
    A. 0.5 volt
    B. 1.0 volt
    C. 1.5 volts
    D. 3.0 volts

50. The contacts of relays and switches used in communication work are frequently silver plated. The purpose of the silver plating is to
    A. improve conductivity of the contacts
    B. reduce arcing at the contacts
    C. improve the flexibility of the contacts
    D. reduce the amount of copper that would otherwise be necessary

KEY (CORRECT ANSWERS)

1.	C	11.	A	21.	C	31.	B	41.	A
2.	A	12.	C	22.	B	32.	A	42.	B
3.	B	13.	D	23.	D	33.	C	43.	B
4.	A	14.	C	24.	B	34.	B	44.	D
5.	C	15.	B	25.	A	35.	C	45.	C
6.	D	16.	D	26.	B	36.	D	46.	D
7.	D	17.	C	27.	D	37.	D	47.	A
8.	D	18.	A	28.	C	38.	C	48.	B
9.	C	19.	D	29.	C	39.	C	49.	D
10.	B	20.	B	30.	D	40.	A	50.	A

TEST 4

DIRECTIONS: Each question or incomplete statement is followed by several suggested answers or completions. Select the one that BEST answers the question or completes the statement. *PRINT THE LETTER OF THE CORRECT ANSWER IN THE SPACE AT THE RIGHT.*

1. If a one microfarad condenser is connected in series with a two microfarad condenser, the capacity of the resulting combination in microfarads is
   A. three
   B. one and one-half
   C. two-thirds
   D. one-third

1.____

2. A storage battery is charged from a 112-volt d-c line through a series resistance.
   If the charging rate is 10 amperes, the electromotive force of the battery is 12 volts and its internal resistance is 0.2 ohms, the value of the series resistance is _____ ohm.
   A. 11.2   B. 10   C. 9.8   D. 1.2

2.____

3. The resistance, in ohms, of a 10 ampere 50M.V shunt is MOST NEARLY
   A. 2   B. .05   C. .005   D. .002

3.____

4. It is required to couple a 4 ohm voice coil of a loudspeaker to an output tube having a plate load of 10,000 ohms. This can best be done by using a transformer having a ratio of primary to secondary turns of APPROXIMATELY
   A. 5   B. 25   C. 50   D. 75

4.____

5. A dynamoelectric amplifier for power control having high amplification ratio is commonly called a(n)
   A. Dynatron
   B. Amplidyne
   C. Amplitherm
   D. Dynatherm

5.____

6. An amplifier has an output voltage wave form that does not exactly follow that of the input voltage. This type of distortion is called _____ distortion.
   A. amplitude   B. modular   C. resonance   D. variation

6.____

7. The frequency in cycles multiplied by 2π is COMMONLY called _____ frequency.
   A. annular   B. heaviside   C. angular   D. circular

7.____

8. An anion is a negative ion that moves toward the
   A. anode in an electrolytic cell
   B. cathode in a discharge tube
   C. positive terminal of a battery while being discharged
   D. negative terminal of a battery while being charged

8.____

2 (#4)

9. Silicon rectifiers, as compared with selenium rectifiers of the same physical size, have
   A. greater current ratings
   B. smaller current ratings
   C. the same current ratings
   D. much greater resistance at 60 cycles

   9.____

10. The germanium rectifier, as compared with other types of rectifiers, has
    A. a high forward drop
    B. a low reverse resistance
    C. no aging, and therefore has an indefinitely long life
    D. a narrow temperature range, from -5° to +40°C

    10.____

11. Transistors are ideally suited for Hi-Fi amplifiers since they are inherently _____ devices.
    A. high impedance
    B. low impedance
    C. non-linear
    D. quadrature

    11.____

12. An air condenser composed of two parallel flat plates of area Z, separated by a distance Y, has a capacitance which is
    A. directly proportional to the distance Y
    B. directly proportional to the area Z
    C. inversely proportional to the area Z
    D. inversely proportional to the square of the area Z

    12.____

13. For audio frequency amplifiers used for Hi-Fi work, it is desirable to have a hum and noise level, at full output, of APPROXIMATELY _____ db.
    A. -80
    B. -20
    C. +20
    D. +80

    13.____

14. The maximum Q of cavity resonators is APPROXIMATELY
    A. 500
    B. 5,000
    C. 50,000
    D. 5,000,000

    14.____

15. To find out if a source of supply is D.C. or A.C., it is BEST to use a(n)
    A. iron vane voltmeter
    B. neon tester
    C. test set made up of two ordinary lamps in series
    D. dynamometer-type voltmeter

    15.____

16. A vacuum tube circuit having high input impedance, low output impedance, and a gain of less than unit is MOST likely a(n) _____ circuit.
    A. anode-follower
    B. differentiating
    C. ignitron
    D. cathode-follower

    16.____

17. A heart-shaped pattern obtained as the response or radiation characteristic of certain directional antennae or as the response characteristic of certain microphones is called a
    A. cardioid pattern
    B. sinusoidal pattern
    C. semicircular pattern
    D. parabolic

    17.____

18. A standard FM broadcast transmitter sends out a signal with a swing of ±60 kc. The percentage modulation of this signal is
    A. 60   B. 70   C. 80   D. 90

19. A standard method of securing a good signal-to-noise ratio in an FM transmitter is to
    A. keep the filament power low to reduce thermal noise
    B. use pre-emphasis
    C. use squelch circuits
    D. use thermal agitation

20. The process of determining the correct values for different positions of a meter, pointer, or settings of a control is COMMONLY called
    A. adjusting   B. measuring   C. aligning   D. calibrating

Questions 21-23.

DIRECTIONS: Questions 21 through 23, inclusive, are to be answered on the basis of the following diagram.

21. In the standard RMA color code for the value of fixed capacitors, when only three color dots are used, the working voltage is assumed to be
    A. 100   B. 300   C. 500   D. 600

22. In standard RMA color code for the value of fixed capacitors when only three color dots are given, the tolerance is assumed to be _____ percent.
    A. 5   B. 10   C. 15   D. 20

23. With reference to the above figure, the dot marked A represents the
    A. first significant figure
    B. decimal multiplier
    C. working temperature
    D. second significant figure

24. If 1000 watts of power are delivered to an antenna having a resistance of 10 ohms, the antenna current, in amperes, is MOST NEARLY
    A. 3.1   B. 5   C. 7.07   D. 10

25. A quarter-wave (90°) antenna comprised of thin wire without supporting structure and operating at a frequency of 5000 kilocycles, has a physical height of _____ feet.
    A. 24.6   B. 49.2   C. 93.8   D. 98.4

4 (#4)

26. As compared with the series-fed antenna, the shunt-fed antenna
    A. permits the elimination of the base ground
    B. need not have an impedance match with the source for optimum operation
    C. permits the elimination of the base insulator
    D. permits the elimination of all insulators

26.____

27. [circuit diagram: e_{in} through series resistor, shunt capacitor, series resistor, shunt capacitor to e_{out}]

    The above diagram represents a(n)
    A. differentiating circuit   B. high pass filter
    C. integrating circuit   D. band pass filter

27.____

28. Of the following, the type of bridge used for measuring inductance is the _____ Bridge.
    A. Kelvin   B. Wheatstone   C. Maxwell   D. Newton

28.____

29. A certain circuit having an input of one volt and an output of 10 volts has a power gain, in decibels, of
    A. 5   B. 10   C. 15   D. 20

29.____

30. In an A.M. transmitter, if the peak value of the modulated carrier current is 2 amps and that of the unmodulated carrier current is one amp, the percentage of modulation is APPROXIMATELY
    A. 40%   B. 60%   C. 80%   D. 100%

30.____

31. With reference to vacuum tubes, if the amplification factor is divided by the plate resistance, the result will be a term called
    A. efficiency   B. transconductance
    C. emission   D. sensitivity

31.____

32. An amplifier in which the grid bias and alternating grid are such that plate current in a specific tube flows at all times with essentially linear amplification is called a class _____ amplifier.
    A. A   B. B   C. C   D. AB$_2$

32.____

33. Inverse feedback is used in audio amplifiers to
    A. magnify the amplification
    B. increase the power output
    C. increase the impedance of the loudspeaker
    D. reduce distortion in the output stage

33.____

34. Constant-current inverse feedback is USUALLY obtained by
    A. increasing the value of the capacitor across the cathode resistor
    B. omitting the bypass capacitor across the cathode tube
    C. increasing the gain of the output tube
    D. decreasing the plate resistance of the output tube

34.____

35. In order to make more natural the reproduction of music which has a very large volume range in a phonograph amplifier, it is BEST to use a(n)
    A. linear response amplifier
    B. volume suppressor
    C. volume expander
    D. output stage with two tubes in push-push

36. The limiter in FM receivers has the function of eliminating _____ from the input to the detector.
    A. the second harmonic
    B. the third harmonic
    C. FM-variations
    D. amplitude variations

Questions 37-39.

DIRECTIONS: Questions 37 through 39 are to be answered on the basis of the following diagram.

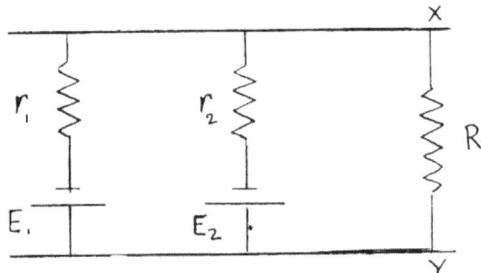

37. If r_1 = .01 ohm, r_2 = .01 ohm, E_1 = 1 volt, and R = infinity, the voltage across xy is MOST NEARLY
    A. 2 volts   B. 1 volt   C. .2 volt   D. .1 volt

38. If r_1 = .01 ohm, r_2 = .01 ohm, E_1 = 1 volt, E_2 = 2 volts, and R = infinity, the voltage across xy is MOST NEARLY
    A. .5   B. 1   C. 1.5   D. 2

39. If r_1 = .01 ohm, r_2 = .01 ohm, E_1 = 1 volt, E_1 = 1 volt, E_2 = 2 volts, and R = 1 ohm, the voltage across xy is MOST NEARLY
    A. .5   B. 9   C. 1.1   D. 1.5

40.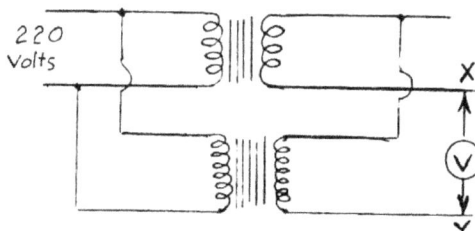

Two transformers with ratios of 2:1 are to be connected in parallel. To test for proper connections, the circuit shown above is used. The transformers may be connected in parallel by connecting Lead "X" to Lead "Y" if the voltmeter shown reads
    A. zero   B. 120   C. 220   D. 340

Questions 41-42.

DIRECTIONS: Questions 41 and 42 are to be answered on the basis of the following figure.

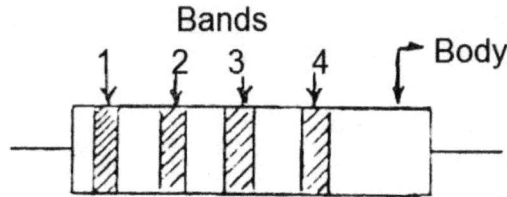

41. In the standard RMA color code chart for the value of resistors, the band numbered 1 in the above figure represents the
    A. decimal multiplier
    B. tolerance
    C. first significant figure
    D. second significant figure

42. With reference to the RMA color code chart for the value of resistors, if the 1st band is red, the 2nd band black, the 3rd band black, and the 4th band silver, the value of this resistor is
    A. 100 ohms 10%
    B. 2000 ohms 5%
    C. 100 ohms 5%
    D. q200 ohms 10%

43. A condenser having a capacitance of one microfarad is connected across a 1000-volt D-C line. The energy stored by this condenser is
    A. 10 watts   B. ½ watt   C. 10 joules   D. ½ joule

44. If a powdered iron core is inserted into an inductance coil, the coil
    A. resistance is increased
    B. inductance is increased
    C. inductance is decreased
    D. resistance is decreased

45. If a brass core is inserted into an inductance coil, the coil
    A. resistance is increased
    B. inductance is increased
    C. inductance is decreased
    D. resistance is decreased

46. A disadvantage of the limiter commonly used in FM receivers is that it requires, for proper operation, a
    A. small signal amplitude
    B. low radio frequency amplification
    C. large signal amplitude
    D. high screen voltage

47. In the ratio detector the radio frequency is fed to the diodes in the same manner as in the FM discriminator except that the diodes in the ratio detector are connected in
    A. parallel   B. push-push   C. push-pull   D. series

48. A general-purpose instrument that may be used for the measurement of the output frequency of an r-f oscillator within accuracies of from .25% to 2% is known as a(n)
    A. absorption wave meter
    B. Wien frequency bridge
    C. Maxwell Bridge
    D. meteorograph bridge

49. The frequency of oscillation of a multivibrator is determined by the values of the
    A. resistance and inductance
    B. inductance and capacity
    C. resistance and capacity
    D. capacity alone

49._____

50. With reference to radio-frequency measurements, a primary standard of frequency is defined as one whose frequency is determined
    A. directly in terms of time
    B. by comparison with another standard
    C. by the value of the RC constant
    D. by the values of L and C in the circuit

50._____

51. If a .75 kw transmitter produces a field intensity of 10 millivolts per meter at a distance of 5 miles and is received by an antenna having an effective height of 10 meters, the millivolts of signal induced in the antenna (neglecting losses) will be MOST NEARLY
    A. 50
    B. 75
    C. 100
    D. 125

51._____

52. With reference to directive microwave antennae, the parabolic reflector possesses the characteristic that
    A. the intensity of the reflected rays varies as the square of the distance
    B. all rays from the radiator striking the reflecting surface are reflected as parallel rays
    C. the intensity of the reflected rays varies inversely as the square of the distance
    D. all rays striking the reflecting surface are reflected as diverging rays

52._____

53. With reference to the oscilloscope, Lissajous curves are widely used for
    A. aligning radio I.F. transformers
    B. aligning television tuners
    C. obtaining a response curve of the I.F. stages in FM receivers
    D. frequency comparison

53._____

54. The one of the following oscillators which is used to deflect periodically the electron beam of a cathode-ray tube so as to give a displacement that is a function of time is the _____ oscillator.
    A. sweep
    B. beat
    C. jump
    D. connecting

54._____

55. The impedance in ohms measured between the terminals of a transmission line at the operating frequency is called _____ impedance.
    A. patch
    B. lumped
    C. surge
    D. sweep

55._____

56. Decibels may be calculated by multiplying the common logarithm of the power ratio by ten. Therefore, a power ratio of 100 corresponds to MOST NEARLY
    A. 10 db
    B. 20 db
    C. 30 db
    D. 40 db

56._____

8 (#4)

57. Power factor is defined as the ratio of active power to apparent power, generally expressed in percent. In accordance with the definition given above, the power factor of a pure resistance is
    A. zero   B. unity   C. infinity   D. indeterminate

Questions 58-59.

DIRECTIONS: Questions 58 and 59 are to be answered on the basis of the following data.

An L resistance attenuation network is required to match, with minimum less, a 500-ohm source Z_S and a 250-ohm lead Z_L; use the design data given below.

$$R_1 = \sqrt{Z_S(Z_S - Z_L)}$$
$$R_2 = \frac{Z_S Z_L}{R_1}$$

58. Using the above data and formula, the value of resistor R_1 for this network is MOST NEARLY
    A. 353   B. 305   C. 253   D. 75

59. With reference to the above L pad and formula, the value of R_2 is MOST NEARLY
    A. 353   B. 305   C. 253   D. 75

60. In frequency modulation receivers, noise
    A. causes an amplitude disturbance only
    B. is completely eliminated by the limiter
    C. causes some variation in the frequency swing of the desired signal
    D. has no effect

61. An open quarter-wave stub may be used as a
    A. suppressor of even and odd harmonics
    B. suppressor of even harmonics only
    C. suppressor of odd harmonics only
    D. filter of odd harmonics only

62. A closed quarter-wave stub offers an infinite impedance at
    A. low frequencies   B. high frequencies
    C. the resonant frequency   D. all frequencies

63. The one of the following which is COMMONLY used as a standing wave detector operating as a current indicator is a _____ pick-up loop with the ends connected to a _____ galvanometer.
    A. one-turn; r-f thermo   B. one-turn; D'Arsonval
    C. 1000-turn; r-f thermo   D. 1000-turn; D'Arsonval

9 (#4)

64. If a line having a characteristic impedance of 300 ohms is terminated in a resistive load of 50 ohms, the standing-wave ratio is MOST NEARLY
 A. 1 to 12 B. 12 to 1 C. 1 to 6 D. 6 to 1

64.____

65. In aligning the sound discriminator of an FM receiver with an oscilloscope, the pattern that should be obtained for proper adjustment is a(n) _____ curve.
 A. symmetrical "S"   B. asymmetrical "S"
 C. symmetrical parabolic   D. asymmetrical parabolic

65.____

66. In AM radio telephone transmitters, negative feedback
 A. is not used
 B. makes impractical the use of high-efficiency systems
 C. makes impractical the use of a power supply system with relatively inexpensive filtering
 D. decreases the amplitude distortion

66.____

Questions 67-70.

DIRECTIONS: Questions 67 through 70 are to be answered on the basis of the following description of a certain transmitter.

The radio transmitter is a frequency-modulated unit utilizing the phase-shift method of obtaining frequency deviations, and as such exhibits considerably different characteristics than the usual amplitude-modulated units.

Intelligence is conveyed in frequency variations of the constant-amplitude carrier wave. The use of the phase-shift method of frequency modulation allows direct crystal control of the mean carrier frequency a necessity in unattended and mobile equipment. It necessitates, however, considerable frequency multiplication after the tubes are used for this function, and a total frequency multiplication of 48 times is effected. A twin triode acts as both crystal oscillator and phase modulator. The first half of the tube operates in a resistance coupled aperiodic oscillator circuit. The output frequency range is 152-162 mc.

The second half of the twin triode acts as a phase modulator. The r-f output of the crystal oscillator is impressed on the phase-modulator grid by means of a blocking condenser. The cathode circuit is provided with a large amount of degeneration by an unbypassed cathode resistor. Because of this degeneration feedback, the transconductance of the triode is abnormally low—so low that the plate current is affected about as much by the direct grid-plate capacitance as by the transconductance. The two effects result in plate current vectors almost 180° apart, and the total plate current is the resultant of the two components. In phase it will be about 90° removed from the phase of the voltage impressed on the grid. When audio is impressed on the grid thereby periodically changing the bias, and in consequence the transconductance, the plate current undergoes a periodic change in both amplitude and phase. The amplitude modulation is unimportant, and is removed in the frequency multipliers, but the phase modulation remains and is the essential element of the transmitted signal.

67. With reference to the above information, the crystal frequency will be between
 A. 152 and 162 mc   B. 15.2 and 16.2 mc
 C. 3166.67 and 3375.0 Kc   D. 316.67 and 337.50 Kc

67.____

68. In the second part of the twin triode, the cathode resistor 68._____
    A. is shunted by a large condenser
    B. has no condenser
    C. is shunted by a small condenser
    D. is in series with an electrolytic condenser

69. In this transmitter, frequency multiplication occurs 69._____
    A. after modulation
    B. before modulation
    C. in the phase modulator
    D. in the oscillator circuit

70. With reference to the above information, when the audio is impressed on the grid of the second triode of the twin triode, 70._____
    A. the plate current undergoes a change in amplitude only
    B. the plate current undergoes a change in amplitude and phase
    C. any amplitude modulation is cut off by the transconductance
    D. any phase modulation is eliminated.

KEY (CORRECT ANSWERS)

1.	C	11.	B	21.	C	31.	B	41.	C	51.	C	61.	B
2.	C	12.	B	22.	D	32.	A	42.	D	52.	B	62.	C
3.	C	13.	A	23.	A	33.	D	43.	D	53.	D	63.	A
4.	C	14.	C	24.	D	34.	B	44.	B	54.	A	64.	D
5.	B	15.	B	25.	B	35.	C	45.	C	55.	C	65.	A
6.	A	16.	D	26.	C	36.	D	46.	C	56.	B	66.	D
7.	C	17.	A	27.	C	37.	B	47.	D	57.	B	67.	C
8.	A	18.	C	28.	C	38.	C	48.	A	58.	A	68.	B
9.	A	19.	B	29.	D	39.	D	49.	C	59.	A	69.	A
10.	C	20.	D	30.	D	40.	A	50.	A	60.	C	70.	B

TEST 5

DIRECTIONS: Each question or incomplete statement is followed by several suggested answers or completions. Select the one that BEST answers the question or completes the statement. *PRINT THE LETTER OF THE CORRECT ANSWER IN THE SPACE AT THE RIGHT.*

1. The unit of measure of magnetomotive force is the
   A. gilbert   B. gauss   C. henry   D. mho

2. The figure of merit of a coil or circuit is
   A. $\frac{R}{Z}$ B. $\frac{X_L}{R}$ C. $X_c X_L$ D. $Z = R$

3. The molecular friction produced by the alternating current reversals in a magnetic core material is known as
   A. retentivity
   B. hysteresis
   C. eddy current
   D. counter M.M.F.

4. One horsepower is equal to ____ watts.
   A. 467   B. 647   C. 1646   D. 746

5. The ability of a magnetic material to conduct magnetic lines of force is called
   A. reluctance
   B. conductance
   C. permeability
   D. admittance

6. A small mica condenser marked with three dots as follows—1. Red, 2. Green, 3. Brown—has a capacitance of what value?
   A. 250 mmf   B. 2500 mmf   C. 25 mmf   D. 2.5 mmf

7. If the current through the windings of an electromagnet is constantly increased, the field strength will increase in proportion to the current, up to a certain point, beyond which the field strength will increase only slightly for a further increase in current. This point is called
   A. permeability
   B. saturation
   C. BH curve
   D. phase point

8. Gold band on a resistor indicates a tolerance of
   A. 10%   B. 20%   C. 5%   D. 15%

9. Placing a "permeability slug" into an rf transformer will
   A. decrease the frequency of the ckt.
   B. increase the frequency of the ckt.
   C. decrease the inductance
   D. none of the above

10. What law states that the total current entering a junction in a circuit is equal to the total current leaving that junction?
    A. Lenz's   B. Coulomb's   C. Ohm's   D. Kirchhoff's

11. The MAXIMUM current carrying capacity of a resistor marked "5000 Ohms-200 Watts" is _____ amperes.
    A. 25   B. .2   C. 2   D. 2.5

12. Three condensers of 2 uF, 2 uF, and 4 uF are connected in series. The resulting capacitance of this combination will be _____ uF.
    A. 0.8   B. 8.0   C. 1.6   D. 16

13. In order to obtain the maximum short circuit current from a group of similar cells in a storage battery, they should be connected in
    A. parallel   B. series-parallel
    C. series   D. parallel-series

14.

    I_T equals _____ amp.
    A. .5   B. 5½   C. 2   D. 0

15. A resistor marked as follows—Body: red; Tip: Green; Band or dot: Orange—has a value of how many ohms?
    A. 1400 ohms   B. 36,000 ohms
    C. 25,000 ohms   D. .25 MEG

16. A 10W, 1000 ohm resistor is in parallel with a 100W, 10,000 ohm resistor and a 50W, 20,000 ohm resistor. The HIGHEST permissible line voltage for this combination without exceeding the power ratings of these resistors is
    A. 1,000 volts   B. 10 volts   C. 100 volts   D. 500 volts

17. The fully charged condition of a lead acid storage cell is indicated when a hydrometer reads
    A. 1.080   B. 1.280   C. 1.150   D. 1.500

18. You are called upon to repair, if possible, a storage battery which is discharged and in which the cells are only half full of electrolyte. You should FIRST
    A. fill with a solution of acid and water to 1200 S.G.
    B. fill with plain distilled water and charge
    C. pour out remaining electrolyte and refill with a new solution of water and acid to 1200 S.G.
    D. none of the above—the battery is beyond repair

19. [circuit diagram showing battery, R₁, voltmeter, R₂, R₃ in series]

The voltmeter connected as shown above will read the voltage drop across
   A. R₁   B. R₂   C. R₁ and R₂   D. R₂ and R₃

20. A radio receiver has a power transformer designed to supply 250 volts when operating from a 110-volt, 60-cycle supply line.
    When the primary is connected to a 110-volt D.C. source, the
    A. secondary voltage will decrease
    B. secondary voltage will increase
    C. primary current will decrease
    D. primary current will increase

21. A coupling system that passes certain frequencies and at the same time rejects other frequencies is called
    A. choke   B. phase shifter
    C. filter   D. bypass condenser

22. Audio frequencies lie between
    A. 200 to 200,000 cps   B. 20 to 20,000 cps
    C. 60 to 120 cps   D. 5 to 4,000 cps

23. Vertical sweep circuits may be distinguished from horizontal by their
    A. higher plate voltages   B. larger capacity condensers
    C. greater power ratings on controls   D. lower plate voltages

24. In an inverted amplifier, output is taken from the _____ circuit.
    A. plate   B. cathode   C. control grid   D. shield grid

25. Poor reception on a newly installed commercial television receiver GENERALLY indicates
    A. improper adjustment of I.F. stages
    B. improper adjustment of 8.25 Mc trap
    C. wrong value R-C components in sweep circuits
    D. poor antenna installation

26. The voltage across the output of the discriminator at resonance should
    A. be a maximum
    B. be a minimum
    C. vary between a maximum and a minimum
    D. be a value depending on the signal voltage

27. For optimum operation of an A.F. resistance coupled voltage amplifier using a triode (not considering frequency restrictions), the plate resistor should be
    A. equal to the plate resistance of the tube
    B. equal to the transconductance of the tube
    C. twice the plate resistance of the tube
    D. equal to plate voltage divided by plate current of the tube

28. Peak inverse voltage being delivered to a full wave rectifier with condenser input is equal to r.m.s. of total secondary
    A. X 1.414
    B. X .707
    C. X. 636
    D. plus voltage on condenser

29. In performing a visual alignment, the voltage fed into the stages to be aligned MUST be
    A. amplitude modulated
    B. unmodulated
    C. frequency modulated
    D. demodulated

30. The discriminator in an FM receiver corresponds to the stage in an AM receiver known as the
    A. converter
    B. second detector
    C. output amplifier
    D. preselector

31. A 200 mmfd padder is connected in series with a 400 mmfd tuning condenser. The total MAXIMUM capacity will be _____ mmfd.
    A. 600
    B. 300
    C. 133
    D. 266

32. Shunting a "tank circuit" with an inducftance will make it
    A. respond to a higher frequency
    B. respond to a lower frequency
    C. destroy its oscillatory action
    D. decrease its resistive component

33. Video frequencies in modern television service range from
    A. 15-15,000 cps
    B. 30-3,500 cps
    C. 44-71 mcs
    D. 4.3-12 mcs

34. A superheterodyne is tuned to a desired signal at 1000 Kc. Its conversion oscillator is operating at 1300 Kc. A signal at _____ Kc may cause an image interference.
    A. 300
    B. 900
    C. 1600
    D. 100

35. The plate E of an RF or IF stage is above normal. The screen grid E is above normal. The cathode E is above normal. Trouble PROBABLY is (E = voltage)
    A. open screen dropping resistor
    B. shorted plate loud resistor
    C. open cathode resistor
    D. shorted screen bi-pass condenser

36. Low output voltage from AC/DC power supply may be caused by open
    A. output filter condenser
    B. condenser in power amplifier cathode circuit
    C. condenser on input side of filter
    D. coupling condenser to power amplifier

37. Adjustments in Lelcher-Wires are GENERALLY accomplished by
    A. sliding a shorting-bar along the line
    B. trimming off the ends of the line
    C. placing a variable condenser across the lines
    D. varying the spacing between the lines

38. Local oscillators in FM receivers often have a mica and a ceramic condenser in parallel across the tank. The purpose of this combination is to
    A. increase the "Q" of the circuit
    B. operate the tank at a greater C/L ratio
    C. prevent temperature co-efficient drift
    D. prevent breakdown of condensers

39. A signal reaching the grid of a grid-leak type of limiter, at a peak value greater than the bias on the tube, will PROBABLY cause
    A. lack of linearity in discriminator output
    B. second-harmonic distortion in A.F. output
    C. saturation in the discriminator "S" curve
    D. normal operation of the stage

40. Frequency adjustments in Klystron tubes are GENERALLY made by
    A. sliding a shorting-bar along the lines
    B. mechanically compressing the tube along its length
    C. tuning the pickup loop
    D. changing the grid-bias

41. The second harmonic of 200 meters is _____ meters.
    A. 400   B. 100   C. 800   D. 50

42. To reduce the natural resonant frequency of a Marconi antenna, we may
    A. place an inductance in series with the antenna
    B. place a condenser in series with the antenna
    C. operate the antenna on a harmonic
    D. reduce the physical length of the antenna

43. The length of a ¼ wave vertical radiator for 800 Kc operation should be ABOUT _____ meters.
    A. 200   B. 94   C. 400   D. 367

44. Alignment of a discriminator is BEST checked by
    A. use of an output meter
    B. use of an audio analyzer
    C. use of a vacuum tube voltmeter
    D. ear

45. A line may be kept non-resonant by
    A. terminating the line at its natural impedance
    B. keeping it an even number of ¼ waves long
    C. twisting or transposing the wires
    D. running one conductor inside the other

46. Placing a reflector behind a di-pole antenna makes it
    A. non-directional
    B. directional away from the reflector
    C. directional toward the side on which the reflector is placed
    D. directional toward its end

47. Klystron tubes depend for their action upon
    A. parallel-line tanks connected to the grids
    B. class "C" operation with a TPTG circuit
    C. bunching of electrons in a velocity-electron stream
    D. circular rotation of electrons under a strong magnetic influence

48. Ordinary vacuum tubes are ineffective in UHF circuits because
    A. their plate currents are too high
    B. heater voltages of 6.3V a.c. are impractical at ultra-high frequencies
    C. socket terminals will arc over at UHF
    D. inter-electrode capacities are too high for ultra-high frequencies

49. Wave-guides are NOT used at low frequencies because
    A. long waves cannot be guided
    B. power is too great at low frequencies
    C. their physical size would be impractical
    D. the wavelength of low frequencies is too short

50. The hum frequency of a full wave rectifier is _____ the frequency of the line voltage frequency.
    A. once
    B. twice
    C. three times
    D. four times

KEY (CORRECT ANSWERS)

1.	A	11.	B	21.	C	31.	C	41.	B
2.	B	12.	A	22.	B	32.	A	42.	A
3.	B	13.	A	23.	B	33.	B	43.	B
4.	D	14.	B	24.	B	34.	C	44.	C
5.	C	15.	C	25.	D	35.	C	45.	A
6.	A	16.	C	26.	B	36.	C	46.	B
7.	B	17.	B	27.	C	37.	A	47.	C
8.	C	18.	B	28.	A	38.	C	48.	D
9.	A	19.	D	29.	C	39.	D	49.	C
10.	D	20.	D	30.	B	40.	B	50.	B

EXAMINATION SECTION
TEST 1

DIRECTIONS: Each question or incomplete statement is followed by several suggested answers or completions. Select the one that BEST answers the question or completes the statement. *PRINT THE LETTER OF THE CORRECT ANSWER IN THE SPACE AT THE RIGHT.*

1. Current in a circuit may be increased by
   A. reducing the circuit resistance
   B. connecting two batteries in parallel
   C. decreasing the voltage
   D. increasing the resistance

2. If a transformer has a primary voltage of 120 volts and a step-up ratio of 1 to 4, the secondary voltage will be _____ V.
   A. 30 B. 120 C. 240 D. 480

3. A(n) _____ type of solid-state device is used as a voltage regulator.
   A. silicon-controlled rectifier B. alloy junction diode
   C. Zener diode D. NPN transistor

4. Impedance matching produces the greatest transfer of
   A. voltage B. current C. impedance D. power

5. A yellow-violet-yellow-silver resistor has a value between
   A. 423kΩ and 517kΩ B. 303kΩ and 403kΩ
   C. 4.5MΩ and 5.1MΩ D. 4kΩ and 5kΩ

6. A parallel resonant circuit at resonance will have
   A. maximum circuit impedance
   B. minimum circuit impedance
   C. zero circuit impedance
   D. high impedance at high frequency and low impedance at low frequency

7. In a series resonant circuit, if the X_L is 500 ohms, the X_C is 500 ohms, and the resistance in the coil is 4 ohms, the impedance of this circuit is _____ Ω.
   A. 22 B. 16 C. 8 D. 4

8. If two capacitors of equal value are connected in series, their TOTAL value will
   A. remain the same B. be one-fourth the value of one
   C. be one-half the value of one D. be twice the value of one

9. If a 600-ohm, 1 watt resistor and a 300-ohm, 1-watt resistor are connected in parallel, the equivalent resistance and wattage are
   A. 900Ω, ½ W B. 900, 2W C. 200Ω, ½ W D. 200Ω, 2W

10. Current-measuring instruments must ALWAYS be connected in
    A. parallel with a circuit
    B. series with a circuit
    C. series parallel with a circuit
    D. delta with the shunt

11. What is the HIGHEST voltage that can be read when the meter is set to the 15-volt range?
    A. 0.15V   B. 1.5V   C. 15V   D. 150V

12. A stroboscope is a test instrument used to check
    A. the speed of a phonograph turntable
    B. waveforms in a color receiver
    C. the accuracy of an oscilloscope
    D. voltages with an oscilloscope

13. A bias box is generally necessary when a serviceman is
    A. making a sweep alignment of the IF stages
    B. measuring AGC bias voltages in a receiver
    C. adjusting the kine bias of a color receiver
    D. adjusting the gray-scale tracking of a color receiver

14. A crosshatch generator is used by a serviceman working on a color receiver when he attempts to make a(n)
    A. IF alignment
    B. gray-scale tracking
    C. dynamic convergence
    D. purity adjustment

15. The power supply of line-voltage operated transistor radios USUALLY utilizes
    A. step-up transformers
    B. swinging chokes
    C. autotransformers
    D. step-down transformers

16. What is the Triac? A
    A. gated transistor
    B. gated Diac
    C. diode
    D. gated SCR

17. Which is a TRU$E statement about the SCR (silicon-controlled rectifier)? It
    A. will not stop conducting until its anode voltage is zero
    B. has a control gate which can turn the SCR off after conduction
    C. has a control gate that can turn the SCR on and off
    D. is a diode

18. Direct-drive record changers use DC brushless motors because of their
    A. high starting torque
    B. stability
    C. ability to use electronic speed controls
    D. low cost

19. The major piece of test equipment used in the alignment of an AM receiver is a(n) _____ generator.
    A. dot
    B. audio-modulated RF
    C. square-wave
    D. sawtooth

20. Corona dope is used to
    A. secure tightened nuts
    B. prevent slipping of belts
    C. bond transformer laminations
    D. suppress high-voltage arcing

21. As a safety precaution, what should a repairman do FIRST before removing a color CRT from its mounting?
    A. Degauss the screen
    B. Short the second anode of the CRT to its aquadag coating
    C. Remove the B plus fuses
    D. Remove the high-voltage rectifier

22. When working on a hot line-connected chassis, a serviceman should use
    A. an isolation transformer to prevent shock hazard
    B. grounded chassis instruments to prevent radiation
    C. an AC meter for accuracy
    D. a variac to reduce line voltage

23. Which of the diagrams of power supplies shown below is a voltage doubler?

24. Which of the schematic symbols shown below represents a silicon-controlled rectifier?

25. Negative feedback in an amplifier will cause
    A. increased gain
    B. increased distortion
    C. decreased gain
    D. regeneration

26. In the circuit shown at the right. what is the forward bias of TR₁?
    A. -10V
    B. -1.7V
    C. -0.9V
    D. -0.8V

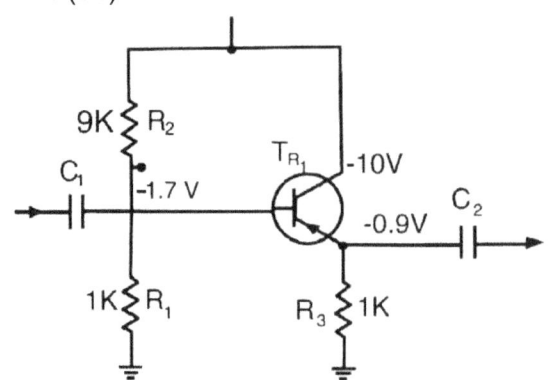

27. Signal feedback from amplifier stages through the power supply is reduced by the use of
    A. decoupling filters
    B. coupling capacitors
    C. blocking capacitors
    D. bandpass filters

28. In a vacuum tube triode, as the grid goes negative, the plate voltage will
    A. decrease toward zero
    B. increase toward B plus
    C. increase, then decrease
    D. remain the same; the grid has no effect

29. The operating characteristics of an FET resemble those of a
    A. junction transistor
    B. Zener diode
    C. triode vacuum tube
    D. pentagrid converter

30. Shorting the emitter to the base of an operating transistor will cause the collector current to
    A. increase
    B. go to zero
    C. remain the same
    D. go to maximum

KEY (CORRECT ANSWERS)

1.	A	11.	C	21.	B
2.	D	12.	A	22.	A
3.	C	13.	C	23.	D
4.	D	14.	C	24.	B
5.	A	15.	D	25.	C
6.	A	16.	D	26.	D
7.	D	17.	A	27.	A
8.	C	18.	C	28.	B
9.	D	19.	B	29.	C
10.	B	20.	D	30.	B

TEST 2

DIRECTIONS: Each question or incomplete statement is followed by several suggested answers or completions. Select the one that BEST answers the question or completes the statement. *PRINT THE LETTER OF THE CORRECT ANSWER IN THE SPACE AT THE RIGHT.*

Questions 1-5.

DIRECTIONS: For each circuit labeled 1 through 5, print in the space at the right the letter of the circuit name chosen from the list below which corresponds to that circuit.

CIRCUITS	CIRCUIT NAMES	
1. 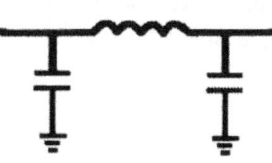	A. Low-pass filter	1.____
	B. Series resonant circuit	
	C. Rumble filter	
2. 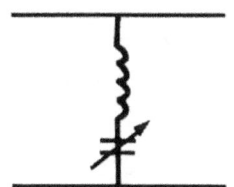	D. Tank circuit	2.____
	E. High-pass filter	
	F. IF transformer	
	G. Piezoelectric filter	
3. 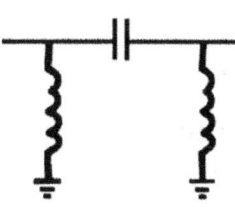		3.____
4. 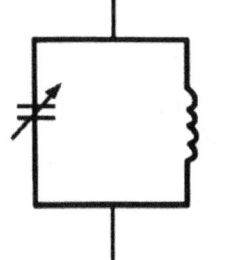		4.____
5. 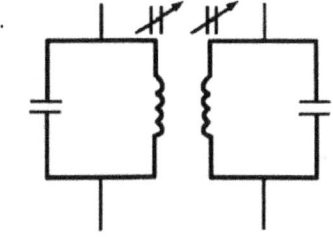		5.____

Questions 6-10.

DIRECTIONS: For each of the meters listed in Items 6 through 10, print in the space at the right the letter of the statement chosen from the list below that BEST characterizes that meter.

METERS	STATEMENTS	
6. VTVM (vacuum tube voltmeter)	A. Measures very small currents	6.____
7. FET (field effect meter)	B. Requires a warm-up period before use	7.____
8. Microammeter (DC)	C. Has very low input impedance	8.____
9. VOM (volt ohmmeter)	D. Input impedance varies with voltage scales	9.____
10. DVM (digital voltmeter	E. Is series connected (AC volts)	10.____
	F. Has very high input impedance	
	G. Is easily read	

Questions 11-15.

DIRECTIONS: For each solid-state device labeled 11 through 15, print in the space at the right the letter of the statement chosen from the list below that BEST characterizes that device.

SOLID-STATE DEVICES STATEMENTS

11.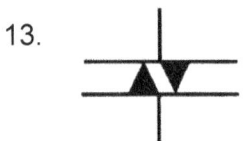

A. It will conduct on positive and negative pulses   11.____

B. It can be destroyed by small static charges   12.____

12.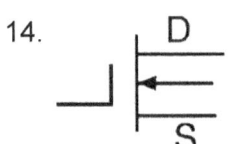

C. It has a low input impedance

D. The gain of this op-amp can be changed easily

13.

E. This FET has a high input impedance, but can be handled safely   13.____

F. The capacity of this varactor can be changed by a DC voltage

14.

G. This diode is wired in the forward-bias position   14.____

15. 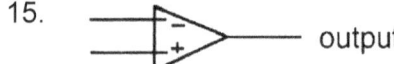 output

5.____

Questions 16-20.

DIRECTIONS: For each of the problems in a tape player listed in Items 16 through 20, print in the space at the right the letter of the defect chosen from the list below that could cause that problem.

PROBLEMS

16. Improper tracking
17. Incorrect tape speed
18. No record – no playback
19. No tape movement
20. Audio distortion

DEFECTS

A. Defective head
B. Burned-out motor
C. Worn belt
D. Oil on braking surface
E. Dirty or magnetized tape head
F. Head out of alignment

16.____
17.____
18.____
19.____
20.____

Questions 21-25.

DIRECTIONS: Questions 21 through 25 are to be answered on the basis of the following diagram.

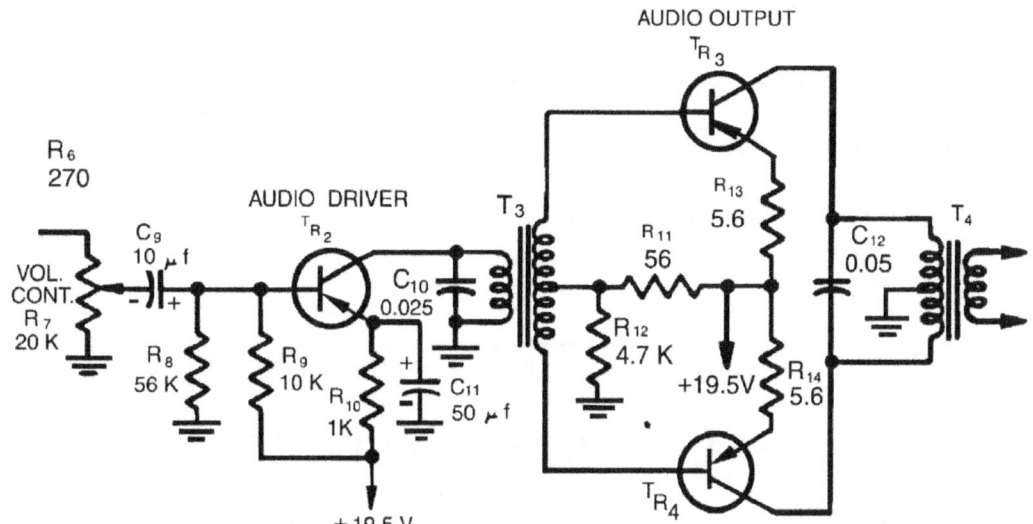

21. What type of transistor is T_{R2}? 21.____

22. Which components provide bias for T_{R2}? 22.____

23. What polarity is the voltage at the collector of T_{R3} as compared to the emitter? 23.____

24. Which component prevents thermal runaway of T_{R4}? 24.____

25. What would happen to the current flowing in T_{R2} if a jumper was connected between its base and emitter?

25.____

Questions 26-30.

DIRECTIONS: Questions 26 through 30 are to be answered on the basis of the following diagram.

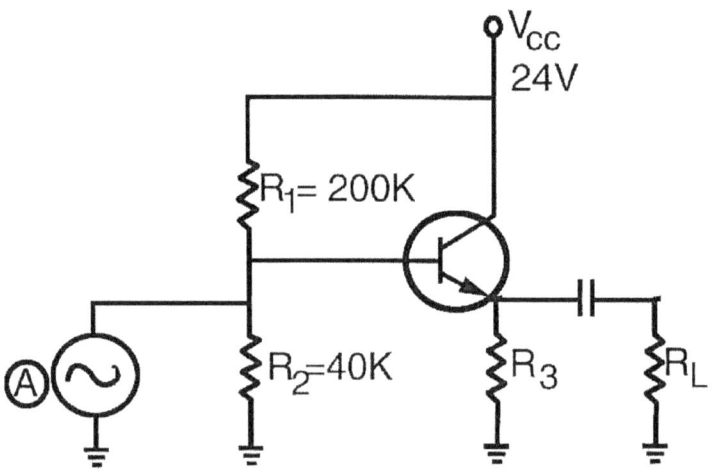

26. Name the circuit drawn. 26.____

27. Calculate the voltage from base to ground. 27.____

28. Name two characteristics of the circuit. 28.____

29. Name one possible purpose for this circuit. 29.____

30. What is Figure A? 30.____

KEY (CORRECT ANSWERS)

1.	A	11.	F	21.	PNP
2.	B	12.	E	22.	$R_8 R_9$
3.	E	13.	A	23.	Negative
4.	D	14.	B	24.	R_{14}
5.	F	15.	D	25.	Goes to zero
6.	B	16.	F	26.	emitter follower
7.	F	17.	D	27.	4 volts
8.	A	18.	B	28.	unity volt gain low out impedance
9.	D	19.	C	29.	drive low impedance RL load
10.	G	20.	E	30.	noise generator (amplifier)

EXAMINATION SECTION
TEST 1

DIRECTIONS: Each question or incomplete statement is followed by several suggested answers or completions. Select the one that BEST answers the question or completes the statement. *PRINT THE LETTER OF THE CORRECT ANSWER IN THE SPACE AT THE RIGHT.*

1. The purpose of the baffle is to   1.____

    A. reduce audible hum
    B. improve low frequency response
    C. increase speaker output response
    D. increase high frequency response

2. A normally operating NPN common emitter transistor has the GREATEST voltage drop between   2.____

    A. emitter and collector   B. base and collector
    C. base and emitter   D. collector and base

3. Heat applied to an operating transistor will   3.____

    A. increase transistor conduction
    B. decrease transistor conduction
    C. improve the PN junction
    D. increase battery life

4. When a superheterodyne receiver with an IF of 455 Khz is tuned to a station of 1010 Khz, the frequency of the local oscillator should be _____ Khz.   4.____

    A. 455   B. 1010   C. 555   D. 1465

5. The complaint about a radio-phono combination set is that it fades on both radio and phono operation.
It is safe to assume that the trouble is   5.____

    A. in the IF amplifier
    B. in the audio amplifier
    C. a faulty converter tube
    D. in the RF amplifier

6. If the screen grid in a power amplifier glows red, it is PROBABLY caused by a(n)   6.____

    A. shorted voice coil
    B. open output transformer
    C. shorted plate bypass
    D. open screen resistor

7. The DC voltage at the rectifier output is zero. The AC input voltage at each plate of the 5Y3 rectifier tube is 250 volts.
This indicates   7.____

    A. a shorted choke
    B. a blown fuse

63

C. defective rectifier tube
D. open output filter capacitor

8. A radio receiver has a loud hum which is not affected by the setting of the volume control. The trouble is PROBABLY caused by

   A. an open volume control
   B. gassy output tube
   C. improper IF alignment
   D. open filter capacitor

9. A speaker designed to reproduce high audio frequencies is called a

   A. woofer
   B. magnetic speaker
   C. PM speaker
   D. tweeter

10. If two .02 Mfd. 400 volt capacitors are connected in series, they are better than one .01 Mfd. 600 volt unit because the two capacitors together will

    A. have more capacity
    B. have a higher coulomb rating
    C. cost less
    D. have a higher voltage rating

11. If tubes in a receiver are connected in series, the tubes must have the same

    A. heater voltage rating
    B. plate voltage
    C. heater current rating
    D. grid bias

12. A resistor is color coded red-red-silver. Its value is _____ ohms.

    A. 22   B. .22   C. 220   D. 2.2

13. If we know the direction of electron flow through a resistor, we

    A. know the amount of voltage across the resistor
    B. are sure the resistor is in good condition
    C. know the value of resistance
    D. know the polarity of the voltage across the resistor

14. The forward resistance of a good semiconductor diode NORMALLY ranges between

    A. 40 and 100 ohms
    B. 1000 and 3500 ohms
    C. one megohm and 3 megohms
    D. ten megohms to infinity

15. A reading of 20 ohms across the primary of an AM IF transformer indicates

    A. winding is shorted
    B. capacitor is shorted
    C. primary is normal
    D. winding is open

16. A line isolation transformer is used to

    A. increase sensitivity
    B. protect a hot chassis from ground
    C. get more volume
    D. decrease hum

17. A limiter is ALWAYS used with _____ detector.   17.____

    A. ratio   B. grid leak
    C. Foster-Seeley   D. gated beam

18. To check for local oscillator operation in a superheterodyne, connect a VTVM from   18.____

    A. oscillator anode to ground
    B. oscillator grid to cathode
    C. converter plate to ground
    D. cathode to ground

19. Positive feedback is used in   19.____

    A. audio amplifiers   B. oscillators
    C. amplifiers   D. mixers

20. The drive capstan is found in   20.____

    A. stereo amplifier   B. tape recorder
    C. multiplex adapters   D. preamplifiers

21. Transistors are damaged by   21.____

    A. heat   B. vibration
    C. high heater voltage D. too little negative bias

22. A heat sink   22.____

    A. heats up the cathodes
    B. removes heat from a power transistor
    C. shields the power supply
    D. insulates the chassis

23. The frequency range of the FM band is   23.____

    A. 60 to 75 Mhz   B. 88 to 108 Mhz
    C. 550 to 1650 Khz   D. 455 to 456 Khz

24. When the bias voltage of a tube is increased,   24.____

    A. plate current goes down
    B. the tube overheats
    C. the tube amplifies more
    D. the cathode current goes up

25. The resistance check of a silicon rectifier in good condition should read   25.____

    A. low resistance in both directions
    B. high resistance in one direction, low resistance in the other
    C. high resistance in both directions
    D. zero in both directions

KEY (CORRECT ANSWERS)

1. B		11. C
2. B		12. D
3. A		13. D
4. D		14. A
5. B		15. C
6. D		16. B
7. C		17. A
8. D		18. A
9. D		19. B
10. D		20. B

21. A
22. B
23. B
24. A
25. B

TEST 2

DIRECTIONS: Each question or incomplete statement is followed by several suggested answers or completions. Select the one that BEST answers the question or completes the statement. *PRINT THE LETTER OF THE CORRECT ANSWER IN THE SPACE AT THE RIGHT.*

1. The property of a coil which opposes current changes is called   1.____

    A. inductance   B. capacitance
    C. resistance   D. conductance

2. The limiter in an FM receiver   2.____

    A. demodulates
    B. is used with a ratio detector
    C. cuts down noises
    D. is found in all FM receivers

3. A push-pull circuit is used to   3.____

    A. double the frequency range that can be handled
    B. increase the harmonic content
    C. cancel out even harmonics, reduce hum, and increase power output
    D. increase total harmonic content and increase power output

4. A limiter tube in an FM receiver is operated   4.____

    A. with the plate at zero B+
    B. without a screen by-pass capacitor
    C. with low plate and screen voltages
    D. with large cathode resistors

5. The current flowing in the emitter circuit of a transistor consists of _____ current.   5.____

    A. collector   B. base
    C. base and collector   D. collector minus the base

6. Two 100 ohm, 10 watt resistors are connected in parallel. The net resistance and power rating will be ohms at _____ watts.   6.____

    A. 200; 5   B. 50; 10   C. 100; 20   D. 50; 20

7. The coupling capacitor between the grid of the output tube and the plate of the voltage amplifier   7.____

    A. blocks DC and allows AC to pass through
    B. allows only DC to pass through
    C. blocks RF and audio frequency signals
    D. blocks RF

8. If the emitter-base forward bias of a transistor increases, the   8.____

    A. emitter current remains constant
    B. collector current decreases

67

C. base current approaches cutoff
D. emitter current increases

9. The base section of an NPN silicon transistor is

   A. formed by fusing N and P type silicon
   B. made of N type silicon
   C. made of P type silicon
   D. made of an insulator

10. Normal base to emitter bias of a germanium transistor used as an amplifier is

    A. 0.2 volt
    B. 2.0 volts
    C. more than 3 volts
    D. negative

11. The terminals of a junction FET are known as the

    A. emitter, base, and collector
    B. anode, cathode, and gate
    C. grid, cathode, and plate
    D. source, drain, and gate

12. What type of solid state device is the BEST replacement for a voltage regulator tube? A(n)

    A. silicon controlled rectifier
    B. alloy junction diode
    C. Zener diode
    D. NPN transistor

13. The majority of current carriers in an N-channel FET are

    A. protons B. holes C. electrons D. ions

14. A grounded emitter transistor amplifier is MOST NEARLY like a _____ amplifier.

    A. grounded grid
    B. grounded cathode
    C. power
    D. triode tube

15. When the cathode of a vacuum tube is heated, it gives off

    A. protons B. electrons C. neutrons D. atoms

16. The base of a transistor is *similar* to a vacuum tube's

    A. plate B. screen C. cathode D. grid

17. The plate current of a 6V6 tube is 38 MA. The screen current is 2 MA. The cathode resistor is 300 ohms.
    The CORRECT bias will be

    A. 18V B. 14V C. 24V D. 12V

18. The MOST commonly used type of radio loudspeaker is

    A. electrodynamic
    B. electrostatic
    C. electromagnetic
    D. PM

19. The name of the stage that obtains audio from a modulated RF signal is called   19.____
    A. audio amplifier   B. RF amplifier
    C. detector   D. oscillator

20. A ratio detector is a type of FM detector that eliminates the need for the following stage,   20.____
    A. audio amplifier   B. rectifier
    C. limiter   D. IF amplifier

21. The point on the tube characteristic curve at which current stops flowing is called   21.____
    A. saturation   B. cut-off
    C. linear portion   D. curved portion

22. The symbol for impedance is   22.____
    A. R   B. E   C. Z   D. I

23. The band width in the IF amplifier of an AM broadcast receiver is   23.____
    A. 10 Khz   B. 5 Khz   C. 3 Mhz   D. 1 Mhz

24. A power transistor is always mounted on a piece of metal so that the metal can act as the   24.____
    A. heat sink   B. base bias
    C. emitter bias   D. spark bias

25. The length of an FM antenna is determined by   25.____
    A. frequency received   B. material used
    C. IF input   D. the audio band

KEY (CORRECT ANSWERS)

1.	A	11.	D
2.	D	12.	C
3.	D	13.	C
4.	A	14.	B
5.	C	15.	B
6.	D	16.	D
7.	A	17.	D
8.	D	18.	D
9.	A	19.	C
10.	A	20.	C

21. B
22. C
23. B
24. A
25. A

TEST 3

DIRECTIONS: Each question or incomplete statement is followed by several suggested answers or completions. Select the one that BEST answers the question or completes the statement. *PRINT THE LETTER OF THE CORRECT ANSWER IN THE SPAE AT THE RIGHT.*

1. A stereo amplifier has _____ channel(s).

   A. 1
   C. 3
   B. 2
   D. none of the above

2. A discriminator in an FM receiver is preceded by

   A. oscillator
   C. mixer
   B. audio amplifier
   D. limiter

3. 1000 milliamperes is equivalent to _____ ampere(s).

   A. .001   B. .1   C. 1   D. 10

4. To widen the trace on an oscilloscope, adjust the _____ control.

   A. vertical amplifier
   C. vertical positioning
   B. horizontal amplifier
   D. horizontal positioning

5. The cathode bypass capacitor is used to

   A. reduce the cathode current
   B. keep the grid voltage constant
   C. isolate the cathode from ground
   D. by-pass the DC voltage to ground

6. A rectifier will

   A. pass current in both directions
   B. change DC to AC
   C. pass current in one direction only
   D. carry high current

7. The process by which a transistor or vacuum tube increases the strength of a signal is known as

   A. regeneration
   C. amplification
   B. degeneration
   D. oscillation

8. Push pull audio circuit tubes are USUALLY operated Class

   A. A   B. B or AB   C. C   D. D

9. The phase inverter circuit supplies the push pull circuit with two signals

   A. in phase
   C. 270° out of phase
   B. 90° out of phase
   D. 180° out of phase

10. 180 PF is equal to _____ MFD.

    A. .00000018   B. .00018   C. 1800   D. 180000

11. The elements of a transistor are 11.____

    A. base collector grid B. plate grid screen
    C. base plate emitter D. emitter base collector

12. The power output of a push pull circuit is 12.____

    A. equivalent to two output tubes in parallel
    B. equivalent to two output tubes in series
    C. greater than two output tubes in parallel
    D. greater than two output tubes in series

13. Pre-amplifiers are needed with a magnetic pickup because 13.____

    A. the pick-up output voltage is too weak
    B. the more tubes you use, the more things can go wrong
    C. it sounds impressive
    D. the pickup output voltage is too strong

14. Sawtooth generator circuits produce the scanning raster, but the sync pulses are needed for 14.____

    A. linearity B. timing
    C. keystoning D. line pairing

15. The raster is tilted with respect to the screen. To straighten the raster, you can adjust the 15.____

    A. ion trap magnet B. picture tube position
    C. focus magnet D. deflection yoke

16. A kinescope brightener 16.____

    A. boosts anode voltage about 10%
    B. boosts heater voltage about 15%
    C. improves secondary emission from grid #2
    D. increases the anode capacitance

17. Black in the reproduced picture corresponds to 17.____

    A. grid-cathode voltage equal to zero
    B. grid-cathode voltage negative at cut-off
    C. minimum anode voltage
    D. average beam current equal to 1 MA

18. An advantage of a silicon diode compared with the 5U4 rectifier tube is 18.____

    A. higher peak inverse voltage rating
    B. higher temperature rating
    C. high forward resistance
    D. smaller size

19. A transformerless power supply has

    A. a voltage doubler and series heaters
    B. a voltage doubler and parallel heaters
    C. a full-wave rectifier and parallel heaters
    D. one side of the power line connected to B+

20. In the flyback high voltage supply,

    A. ripple frequency is 60 c.p.s.
    B. a full-wave rectifier is used
    C. the HV rectifier filament can be in a series string with all other tubes
    D. the sharp drop in horizontal output current produces the AC high voltage

21. With an open 3/8 amp. fuse in the high voltage case, the result will be

    A. no brightness, normal sound
    B. no brightness, no sound
    C. normal raster, no heaters, light
    D. small raster, weak sound

22. The composite video signal for the video amplifier is obtained from the

    A. video detector
    B. sound IF section
    C. kinescope cathode
    D. RF tuner

23. The video amplifier gain determines

    A. brightness
    B. contrast
    C. resolution
    D. detail

24. Which stage is NOT necessary for producing horizontal output?

    A. Horizontal oscillator
    B. Damper
    C. Horizontal amplifier
    D. Horizontal AFC

25. When the horizontal amplifier is conducting peak plate current, the electron scanning beam is at the

    A. left edge of the raster
    B. right edge of the raster
    C. center of trace
    D. center of flyback

KEY (CORRECT ANSWERS)

1. B
2. D
3. C
4. B
5. C

6. C
7. C
8. B
9. D
10. B

11. D
12. B
13. A
14. B
15. D

16. B
17. B
18. D
19. D
20. D

21. A
22. A
23. C
24. B
25. B

———

TEST 4

DIRECTIONS: Each question or incomplete statement is followed by several suggested answers or completions. Select the one that BEST answers the question or completes the statement. *PRINT THE LETTER OF THE CORRECT ANSWER IN THE SPACE AT THE RIGHT.*

1. The ion-trap magnet is adjusted for

   A. minimum brightness B. maximum brightness
   C. maximum deflection D. proper centering

2. Current in the deflection coils for horizontal scanning provides magnetic field lines that are _____ the beam.

   A. circular around
   B. horizontal above and below
   C. vertical left and right of
   D. parallel to

3. The ripple frequency of a half wave voltage doubler is _____ cps.

   A. 60   B. 120   C. 240   D. 30

4. If the kinescope DC cathode voltage is +120 volts, for -30 volts of grid bias, the grid voltage is _____ volts.

   A. -30   B. +30   C. +90   D. +150

5. The top of the picture is stretched with too much raster height. To correct this,

   A. vary the vertical hold control
   B. reduce height with vertical linearity control
   C. increase height with size control
   D. replace vertical oscillator tube

6. The frequency of the sawtooth plate current in the horizontal amplifier is _____ cps.

   A. 60   B. 10,500   C. 15,750   D. 5,750

7. Retraces are NOT visible because of _____ pulses.

   A. synchronizing B. vertical
   C. horizontal   D. blanking

8. To eliminate ghosts in the picture,

   A. use a longer transmission line
   B. connect a booster
   C. change antenna orientation or location
   D. twist the transmission line

9. Powdered iron cores are GENERALLY used in

   A. power transformers   B. non-inductive resistors
   C. dynamic speakers   D. IF transformers

2 (#4)

10. A resistor having a value of less than 100 ohms is in series with a selenium rectifier to   10.____
    A. improve the filtering action
    B. eliminate hum distortion
    C. prevent current surges from damaging the rectifier
    D. prevent damage to a series filament circuit

11. Hum troubles, when caused by the power supply, are GENERALLY due to the   11.____
    A. power transformer   B. filter capacitor
    C. filter resistor   D. fuse

12. It is BEST to install an FM antenna as high as possible because it   12.____
    A. is less expensive   B. looks impressive
    C. gets strongest signal   D. is less costly

13. The following tube CANNOT be used as an amplifier: 13.____
    A. Diode   B. Triode   C. Tetrode   D. Pentode

14. The reading of resistance between base and emitter in a forward direction should be   14.____
    A. high   B. low
    C. very high   D. none of the above

15. The *wow* in a phonograph reproduction is USUALLY caused by   15.____
    A. a bad needle   B. a cracked crystal
    C. changing motor speed   D. a defective tube

16. After detection, the carrier frequency is eliminated by a   16.____
    A. tube   B. transistor
    C. resistor   D. capacitor

17. Inductance is provided by a   17.____
    A. resistor   B. tube   C. coil   D. capacitor

18. Frequency band width of an FM wave depends upon   18.____
    A. ratio detector
    B. discriminator
    C. RF carrier
    D. strength of the impressed audio voltage

19. Which of the following does NOT affect the chrominance signal?   19.____
    A. Antenna   B. Fine tuning control
    C. Synchronous demodulator D. 4.5 Mhz IF amplifier

20. The output of the chrominance band--pass amplifier   20.____
    A. drives the color reference oscillator
    B. is varied by the hue control
    C. drives the synchronous demodulators
    D. operates the color killer

21. Which of the following applies for a monochrome signal?　　　　21.___

    A. Color amplifier conducting
    B. Color killer conducting
    C. Maximum output from color phase detector
    D. Maximum G-Y video signal

22. To reduce color fringes at the bottom of a monochrome picture, adjust the　　　　22.___

    A. color level control
    B. purity magnet
    C. dynamic convergence
    D. color video drive signals

23. To eliminate the color in the center area of a white raster, adjust the　　　　23.___

    A. purity magnet　　　　　　　　B. hue control
    C. color level control　　　　　D. red screen-grid control

24. If you turn down the blue screen grid control but allow the red and green guns to operate, without a picture you will see　　　　24.___

    A. yellow raster　　　　　　　　B. blue raster
    C. color fringes　　　　　　　　D. diagonal color stripes

25. Which of the following is cut off during horizontal trace time?　　　　25.___

    A. Color amplifier
    B. Sync burst separator
    C. Color reference oscillator
    D. Y video amplifier

KEY (CORRECT ANSWERS)

1.	D	11.	B
2.	C	12.	C
3.	A	13.	A
4.	C	14.	B
5.	B	15.	C
6.	C	16.	D
7.	D	17.	C
8.	C	18.	B
9.	D	19.	D
10.	C	20.	B

21. B
22. D
23. A
24. A
25. B

TEST 5

Questions 1-10.

DIRECTIONS: Select the lettered word or phrase in Column II which matches the numbered item in Column I. *PRINT THE LETTER OF THE CORRECT ANSWER IN THE SPACE AT THE RIGHT.*

COLUMN I

1. bias
2. silicon
3. resonance
4. hertz
5. reactance
6. meters
7. capacitance
8. inductance
9. MU
10. reluctance

COLUMN II

A. suppressor
B. henries
C. pico-farads
D. magnetic
E. ohmmeter
F. amplification factor
G. grid to cathode
H. rectifier
I. cycles per second
J. AC resistance
K. wave length
L. tuned circuit
M. inverse feedback

1.____
2.____
3.____
4.____
5.____
6.____
7.____
8.____
9.____
10.____

Questions 11-20.

DIRECTIONS: Select the lettered word or phrase in Column II which matches the numbered item in Column I. *PRINT THE LETTER OF THE CORRECT ANSWER IN THE SPACE AT THE RIGHT.*

COLUMN I

11. no picture, no sound, no raster
12. horizontal line across screen
13. snowy picture
14. no sound, picture normal
15. picture torn apart in diagonal bars
16. no picture, normal raster and sound
17. overload distortion
18. poor vertical linearity
19. no high voltage
20. low B+

COLUMN II

A. DC bias for CRT
B. small raster
C. horizontal AFC
D. gain level for video signal
E. weak RF signal
F. A G C adjustment
G. weak vertical output tube
H. no brightness
I. defective vertical oscillator
J. 4.5 Mhz–IF amplifier
K. dead low voltage rectifier
L. video amplifier

11.____
12.____
13.____
14.____
15.____
16.____
17.____
18.____
19.____
20.____

Questions 21-30.

DIRECTIONS: Fill in the blank space(s) the word (or words) which is(are) the CORRECT answer(s) to the question.

21. When two equal resistors are connected in parallel, the total resistance will be _____ than one resistor. 21.___

22. .043 amps is equal to _____ MA. 22.___

23. .001 MFD is equal to _____ PF. 23.___

24. A PNP transistor has _____ material in the base. 24.___

25. A circuit used to keep volume levels nearly equal on all station is called _____. 25.___

26. *Motorboating* is usually caused by a(n) _____ second filter capacitor. 26.___

27. Video signal amplitude determines the picture quality called _____. 27.___

28. The bandwidth of a television signal is _____ Mhz. 28.___

29. The type of modulation of the transmitted picture carrier signal is _____. 29.___

30. The type of modulation of the transmitted TV sound carrier signal is _____. 30.___

KEY (CORRECT ANSWERS)

1. G
2. H
3. L
4. I
5. J

6. K
7. C
8. B
9. M
10. D

11. K
12. I
13. E
14. A
15. C

16. L
17. D
18. F
19. H
20. B

21. 1/2
22. 43
23. 1000
24. N
25. AGC

26. open
27. resolution
28. 6
29. frequency
30. amplitude

EXAMINATION SECTION
TEST 1

DIRECTIONS: Each question or incomplete statement is followed by several suggested answers or completions. Select the one that BEST answers the question or completes the statement. *PRINT THE LETTER OF THE CORRECT ANSWER IN THE SPACE AT THE RIGHT.*

1. Two 100 ohm, 10 watt resistors are connected in parallel. The net resistance and power rating will be _____ ohms at _____ watts. 1._____

    A. 200; 5　　　B. 50; 10　　　C. 100; 20　　　D. 50; 20

2. A push-pull circuit is used to 2._____

    A. double the frequency range that can be handled
    B. increase the harmonic content
    C. cancel out even harmonics, reduce hum, and increase power output
    D. increase total harmonic content and increase power output

3. A reading of 20 ohms across the primary of an AM IF transformer indicates 3._____

    A. winding is shorted　　　B. capacitor is shorted
    C. primary is normal　　　D. winding is open

4. The phase inverter circuit supplies the push-pull circuit with two signals _____ phase. 4._____

    A. in　　　B. 90 out of
    C. 270 out of　　　D. 180 out of

5. When a superheterodyne receiver with an IF of 455 Khz is tuned to a station of 1010 Khz, the frequency of the local oscillator should be _____ Khz. 5._____

    A. 455　　　B. 1010　　　C. 555　　　D. 1465

6. Positive feedback is used in 6._____

    A. audio amplifiers　　　B. oscillators
    C. amplifiers　　　D. mixers

7. A resistance check of a silicon rectifier in good condition should read 7._____

    A. low resistance in both directions
    B. high resistance in one direction, low resistance in the other
    C. high resistance in both directions
    D. zero in both directions

8. A crosshatch generator is used by a serviceman working on a color receiver when he attempts to make a(n) 8._____

    A. IF alignment　　　B. gray scale tracking
    C. dynamic convergence　　　D. purity adjustment

9. Current in a circuit may be increased by 9._____

    A. reducing the circuit resistance
    B. connecting two batteries in parallel

81

C. decreasing the voltage
D. increasing the resistance

10. The forward resistance of a good semiconductor diode NORMALLY ranges between 10.___

    A. 40 and 100 ohms
    B. 1000 and 3500 ohms
    C. one megohm and 3 megohms
    D. ten megohms to infinity

11. If we know the direction of electron flow through a resistor, we 11.___

    A. know the amount of voltage across the resistor
    B. are sure the resistor is in good condition
    C. know the value of resistance
    D. know the polarity of the voltage across the resistor

12. A normally operating NPN common emitter transistor has the GREATEST voltage drop between 12.___

    A. emitter and collector   B. base and collector
    C. base and emitter   D. collector and base

13. A rectifier will 13.___

    A. pass current in both directions
    B. change DC to AC
    C. pass current in one direction *only*
    D. carry high current

14. The length of an FM antenna is determined by 14.___

    A. frequency received   B. material used
    C. IF input   D. the audio band

15. 1000 milliamperes is equivalent to _____ amperes. 15.___

    A. .001   B. .1   C. 1   D. 10

16. An inoperative oscillator stage in the tuner will result in 16.___

    A. no raster   B. no picture and no sound
    C. high voltage at the CRT   D. hum bars in the picture

17. A power transistor is ALWAYS mounted on a piece of metal so that the metal can act as the 17.___

    A. heat sink   B. base bias
    C. emitter bias   D. spark bias

18. The frequency range of the FM band is 18.___

    A. 60 to 75 Mhz   B. 88 to 108 Mhz
    C. 550 to 1650 Khz   D. 455 to 456 Khz

19. A Triac is a

    A. gated transistor
    B. gated Diac
    C. diode
    D. gated SCR

20. It is important, when coupling a transistor output to a speaker, to match the

    A. impedance   B. voltage   C. current   D. size

21. The reading of resistance between base and emitter in a forward direction should be

    A. high
    B. low
    C. very high
    D. none of the above

22. If a transformer has primary voltage of 120 volts and a step-up of 1 to 4, the secondary voltage will be _____ V.

    A. 30   B. 120   C. 240   D. 480

23. A yellow-violet-yellow-silver resistor has a value between

    A. 423 K and 517 K
    B. 303 K and 403 K
    C. 4.5 M and 5.1 M
    D. 4 K and 5 K

24. Heat applied to an operating transistor will

    A. increase transistor conduction
    B. decrease transistor conduction
    C. improve the PN junction
    D. increase battery life

25. 180 PF is equal to _____ MFD.

    A. .00000018   B. .00018   C. 1800   D. 18000

KEY (CORRECT ANSWERS)

1. D		11. D	
2. D		12. B	
3. C		13. C	
4. D		14. A	
5. D		15. C	
6. B		16. B	
7. B		17. A	
8. C		18. B	
9. A		19. D	
10. A		20. A	

21. B
22. D
23. A
24. A
25. B

TEST 2

DIRECTIONS: Each question or incomplete statement is followed by several suggested answers or completions. Select the one that BEST answers the question or completes the statement. *PRINT THE LETTER OF THE CORRECT ANSWER IN THE SPACE AT THE RIGHT.*

1. Impedance matching produces the GREATEST transfer of 1.____

   A. voltage   B. current   C. impedance   D. power

2. If two capacitors of equal value are connected in series, their TOTAL value will 2.____

   A. remain the same
   B. be one-fourth the value of one
   C. be one-half the value of one
   D. be twice the value of one

3. The drive capstan is found in 3.____

   A. stereo amplifier   B. tape recorder
   C. multiplex adapters   D. preamplifiers

4. Transistors are damaged by 4.____

   A. heat   B. vibration
   C. high heater voltage   D. too little negative bias

5. A heat sink 5.____

   A. heats up the cathodes
   B. removes heat from a power
   C. shields the power supply
   D. insulates the chassis

6. A solid state device that is the BEST replacement for a voltage regulator tube is a(n) 6.____

   A. silicon controlled rectifier
   B. alloy junction diode
   C. Zener diode
   D. NPN transistor

7. Inductance is provided by a 7.____

   A. resistor   B. tube   C. coil   D. capacitor

8. After detection, the carrier frequency is eliminated by a 8.____

   A. tube   B. transistor
   C. resistor   D. capacitor

9. If a 600 ohm, 1 watt resistor and a 300 ohm, 1 watt resistor are connected in parallel, the equivalent resistance and wattage are _____ and _____ watt(s). 9.____

   A. 900; 1/2   B. 600; 1   C. 400; 4   D. 200; 2

10. If two .02 Mfd, 400 volt capacitors are connected in series, they are better than one .01 Mfd, 600 volt unit because the two capacitors together will

    A. have more capacity
    B. have a higher coulomb rating
    C. cost less
    D. have a higher voltage rating

11. To widen the trace on an oscilloscope, adjust the _____ control.

    A. vertical amplifier   B. horizontal amplifier
    C. vertical positioning   D. horizontal positioning

12. Demodulation takes place in the

    A. AVC   B. audio
    C. detector   D. power supply

13. Which is a TRUE statement about the SCR (silicon-controlled rectifier)? It

    A. will not stop conducting until its anode voltage is zero
    B. has a control gate which can turn the SCR off after conduction
    C. has a control gate that can turn the SCR on and off
    D. is a diode

14. The majority of current carriers in an N-channel FET are

    A. protons   B. holes   C. electrons   D. ions

15. Current-measuring instruments must ALWAYS be connected in

    A. parallel with a circuit
    B. series with a circuit
    C. series parallel with a circuit
    D. delta with the shunt

16. What is the HIGHEST voltage that can be read when the meter is set to the 15 volt range?
    _____ V.

    A. 0.15   B. 1.5   C. 15   D. 150

17. A stroboscope is a test instrument used to check

    A. the speed of a phonograph turntable
    B. waveforms in a color receiver
    C. the accuracy of an oscilloscope
    D. voltages with an oscilloscope

18. A transformerless power supply has

    A. a voltage doubler and series heaters
    B. a voltage doubler and parallel heaters
    C. a full-wave rectifier and parallel heaters
    D. one side of the power line connected to B+

19. When working on a hot line connected chassis, a serviceman should use

    A. an isolation transformer to prevent shock hazard
    B. grounded chassis instruments to prevent radiation
    C. an AC meter for accuracy
    D. a variac to reduce line voltage

20. A resistor having a value of less than 100 ohms is in series with a selenium rectifier to

    A. improve the filtering action
    B. eliminate hum distortion
    C. prevent current surges from damaging the rectifier
    D. prevent damage to a series filament circuit

21. The cathode by-pass capacitor is used to

    A. reduce the cathode current
    B. keep the grid voltage constant
    C. isolate the cathode from ground
    D. by-pass the DC voltage to ground

22. Negative feedback in an amplifier will cause

    A. increased gain
    B. increased distortion
    C. decreased gain
    D. regeneration

23. The top of the picture is stretched with too much raster height.
    To correct this,

    A. vary the vertical hold control
    B. reduce height with vertical linearity control
    C. increase height with size control
    D. replace vertical oscillator tube

24. What type of solid state device is the BEST replacement for a voltage regulator tube?
    A(n)

    A. silicon controlled rectifier
    B. alloy junction diode
    C. Zener diode
    D. NPN transistor

25. The reading of resistance between base and emitter in a forward direction should be

    A. high
    B. low
    C. very high
    D. none of the above

KEY (CORRECT ANSWERS)

1. D
2. C
3. B
4. A
5. B

6. C
7. C
8. D
9. D
10. D

11. B
12. C
13. A
14. C
15. B

16. C
17. A
18. D
19. A
20. C

21. C
22. C
23. B
24. C
25. B

TEST 3

Questions 1-20.

DIRECTIONS: Select the lettered word or phrase in Column II which matches the numbered item in Column I. *PRINT THE LETTER OF THE CORRECT ANSWER IN THE SPACE AT THE RIGHT.*

COLUMN I

1. Rectifier
2. Attenuator
3. Degausse
4. Reactance
5. EMF
6. Anode
7. Dielectric
8. Inductance
9. Mho
10. Potentiometer
11. Detector
12. AM
13. Self excited oscillator
14. Absorption frequency meter
15. Binary
16. Farad
17. Impedance
18. Zener diode
19. Resonance
20. Beta

COLUMN II

A. Voltage
B. Insulator
C. The property of a circuit that opposes any change of current
D. Changes IF to AF of a carrier with an AF signal
E. Amplitude varies
F. Unit of conductance
G. A device that decreases strength
H. Checks frequency of a transmitter
I. Number system using zeros and ones
J. Unit of measurement for capacitors
K. Reducing magnetization to zero
L. Total current opposition in an AC circuit
M. Positively charged electrode toward which electrons flow
N. $X_L = X_C$
O. Current gain in a transistor
P. Changes AC to DC
Q. Reduces arcing
R. Variable resistor
S. Regulates voltage
T. Opposition to AC by a coil or capacitor
U. Metric prefix meaning ten
V. Multiple path circuit
W. Uses a tuned tank in the grid circuit
X. Stores electricity
Y. Variable coil
Z. Increases amplitude

1.___
2.___
3.___
4.___
5.___
6.___
7.___
8.___
9.___
10.___
11.___
12.___
13.___
14.___
15.___
16.___
17.___
18.___
19.___
20.___

Questions 21-35.

DIRECTIONS: Each of the following statements have one or more missing words as indicated by an underline. Write the missing words as indicated by an underline.

21. Kirchhoffs voltage law states that the algebraic sum of all voltages around any closed path must be equal to _____. 21.____

22. An ammeter is always connected in _____ to measure the circuit current. 22.____

23. The amount of charge a capacitor has stored after the first time constant is equal to _____ percent of the applied voltage. 23.____

24. The standard IF frequency in an FM receiver is _____. 24.____

25. A sin-wave AC circuit with XC and R in series, the voltage across R _____ the voltage across XC by 90. 25.____

26. Thin sheets of steel insulated from one another are used to reduce _____ losses in inductors, motors, and transformers. 26.____

27. A device which converts a digital signal to an analog signal is referred to as a _____ converter. 27.____

28. In a radio receiver, the mixing of two signals is referred to as _____. 28.____

29. On a frequency response curve, the bandwidth is measured between the half-power points. At what percentage point is this located? _____. 29.____

30. The ripple frequency of a full wave rectifier is _____. 30.____

31. What transistor configuration would you find if the output is taken off the emitter? _____ 31.____

32. A diode which is used for regulation in a power supply is referred to as a _____ diode. 32.____

33. For maximum power transfer, the load impedance should _____ the impedance of the source. 33.____

34. A diode will conduct only when the cathode is _____ with respect to the anode. 34.____

35. A parallel resonant circuit offers a _____ impedance to its resonant frequency. 35.____

KEY (CORRECT ANSWERS)

1.	P	16.	J
2.	G	17.	L
3.	K	18.	S
4.	T	19.	N
5.	A	20.	O
6.	M	21.	zero
7.	B	22.	series
8.	C	23.	63
9.	F	24.	10.8 Mhz
10.	R	25.	leads
11.	D	26.	eddy current
12.	E	27.	D to A
13.	W	28.	mixing
14.	H	29.	70.7%
15.	I	30.	120 Hz

31. emitter follower
32. zener
33. equal
34. negative
35. high

EXAMINATION SECTION
TEST 1

DIRECTIONS: Each question or incomplete statement is followed by several suggested answers or completions. Select the one that BEST answers the question or completes the statement. *PRINT THE LETTER OF THE CORRECT ANSWER IN THE SPACE AT THE RIGHT.*

1. A normally operating NPN common emitter transistor has the GREATEST voltage drop between

   A. emitter and collector
   B. base and collector
   C. base and emitter
   D. plate and grid

2. When a superheterodyne receiver with an IF of 455 Khz is tuned to a station of 1010 Khz, the frequency of the local oscillator should be _____ Khz.

   A. 455　　　B. 1010　　　C. 555　　　D. 1465

3. The DC voltage at the rectifier output is zero. The AC input is 125 volts. This indicates

   A. a shorted choke
   B. capacitor is wrong value
   C. defective rectifier tube
   D. open output filter capacitor

4. A radio receiver has a loud hum which is NOT affected by the setting of the volume control.
   The trouble is *probably* caused by

   A. an open volume control
   B. a gassy output tube
   C. improper IF alignment
   D. an open filter capacitor

5. A speaker designed to reproduce high audio frequencies is called

   A. woofer
   B. magnetic speaker
   C. PM speaker
   D. tweeter

6. If two .02 MFd. 400 volt capacitors are connected in series, they are better than one .01MFd. 600 volt unit because the two capacitors together will

   A. have more capacity
   B. have a higher coulomb rating
   C. cost less
   D. have a higher voltage rating

7. Powdered iron cores are *generally* used in

   A. power transformers
   B. non-inductive resistors
   C. dynamic speakers
   D. IF transformers

8. A resistor having a value of less than 100 ohms is in series with a selenium rectifier to   8.___

   A. improve the filtering action
   B. eliminate hum distortion
   C. prevent current surges from damaging the rectifier
   D. prevent damage to a series filament circuit

9. Hum troubles, when caused by the power supply, are *generally* due to the   9.___

   A. power transformer   B. filter capacitor
   C. filter resistor   D. fuse

10. The ripple frequency of a half wave voltage doubler is _____ cps.   10.___

    A. 60   B. 129   C. 240   D. 30

11. Pre-amplifiers are needed with a magnetic pickup because   11.___

    A. the pick-up output voltage is too weak
    B. the more tubes you use, the more things can go wrong
    C. it sounds impressive
    D. the pick-up output voltage is too strong

12. A transformerless power supply has   12.___

    A. a voltage doubler and series heaters
    B. a voltage doubler and parallel heaters
    C. a full-wave rectifier and parallel heaters
    D. one side of the power line connected to B+

13. After detection, the carrier frequency is eliminated by a   13.___

    A. tube   B. transistor   C. resistor   D. capacitor

14. Inductance is provided by a   14.___

    A. resistor B. tube   C. coil   D. capacitor

15. Frequency band width of an FM wave depends upon   15.___

    A. ratio detector
    B. discriminator
    C. RF carrier
    D. strength of the impressed audio voltage

16. The _____ tube CANNOT be used as an amplifier.   16.___

    A. diode   B. triode   C. tetrode   D. pentode

17. The reading of resistance between base and emitter in a forward direction should be   17.___

    A. high   B. low
    C. very high   D. none of the above

18. A resistor is color coded red-red-silver.   18.___
    Its value is _____ ohms.

    A. 22   B. .22   C. 220   D. 2.2

19. If we know the direction of electron flow through a resistor, we

    A. know the amount of voltage across the resistor
    B. are sure the resistor is in good condition
    C. know the value of resistance
    D. know the polarity of the voltage across the resistor

20. To see a sine wave on an oscilloscope screen, the signal is *generally* injected into the _____ circuit.

    A. horizontal B. high voltage
    C. brightness D. vertical

21. It is important, when coupling a transistor output to a speaker, to match the

    A. impedance   B. voltage   C. current   D. size

22. A line isolation transformer is used to

    A. *increase* sensitivity
    B. protect a hot chassis from ground
    C. get more volume
    D. *decrease* hum

23. Positive feedback is used in

    A. audio amplifiers   B. oscillators
    C. amplifiers   D. mixers

24. Transistors are damaged by

    A. heat   B. vibration
    C. high heater voltage D. too little negative bias

25. A heat sink

    A. heats up the cathodes
    B. removes heat from a power transistor
    C. shields the power supply
    D. insulates the chassis

KEY (CORRECT ANSWERS)

1. B
2. D
3. C
4. D
5. D

6. D
7. D
8. C
9. B
10. A

11. A
12. A
13. D
14. C
15. D

16. A
17. B
18. B
19. D
20. D

21. A
22. B
23. B
24. A
25. B

TEST 2

DIRECTIONS: Each question or incomplete statement is followed by several suggested answers or completions. Select the one that BEST answers the question or completes the statement. *PRINT THE LETTER OF THE CORRECT ANSWER IN THE SPACE AT THE RIGHT.*

1. The frequency range of the FM band is

   A. 60 to 75 Mhz B. 88 to 108 Mhz
   C. 550 to 1650 Khz D. 455 to 456 Khz

2. What type of solid state device is the BEST replacement for a voltage regulator tube?

   A. Silicon controlled rectifier
   B. Alloy junction diode
   C. Zener diode
   D. NPN transistor

3. The MAJORITY of current carriers in an N-channel FET are

   A. protons   B. holes   C. electrons   D. ions

4. A grounded emitter transistor amplifier is *most nearly* like a

   A. grounded grid amplifier
   B. grounded cathode amplifier
   C. power amplifier
   D. triode tube amplifier

5. The base of a transistor is *similar* to a vacuum tube's

   A. plate   B. screen   C. cathode   D. grid

6. The name of the stage that obtains audio from a modulated RF signal is called

   A. audio amplifier B. RF amplifier
   C. detector D. oscillator

7. The point on the tube characteristic curve at which current stops flowing is called

   A. saturation B. cut-off
   C. linear portion D. curved portion

8. The band width in the IF amplifier of an AM broadcast receiver is

   A. 15 Khz   B. 5 Khz   C. 3 Mhz   D. 1 Mhz

9. A power transistor is ALWAYS mounted on a piece of metal so that the metal can act as the

   A. heat sink B. base bias
   C. emitter bias D. spark bias

10. The length of an FM antenna is determined by

    A. frequency received B. material used
    C. IF input D. the audio band

11. 1000 milliamperes is equivalent to _____ amperes.   11.___

    A. .001   B. .1   C. 1   D. 10

12. To widen the trace on an oscilloscope, adjust the _____ control.   12.___

    A. vertical amplifier   B. horizontal amplifier
    C. vertical positioning   D. horizontal positioning

13. A rectifier will   13.___

    A. pass current in both directions
    B. change DC to AC
    C. pass current in one direction only
    D. carry high current

14. The process by which a transistor or vacuum tube *increases* the strength of a signal is known as   14.___

    A. regeneration   B. degeneration
    C. amplification   D. oscillation

15. The phase inverter circuit supplies the push-pull circuit with two signals   15.___

    A. in phase   B. 90° out of phase
    C. 270° out of phase   D. 180° out of phase

16. 180 PF is equal to _____ MFD.   16.___

    A. .00000018   B. .00018   C. 1800   D. 180000

17. The element of a transistor is the   17.___

    A. base collector grid   B. plate grid screen
    C. base plate emitter   D. emitter base collector

18. A resistance check of a silicon diode in good condition should read   18.___

    A. *low* resistance in both directions
    B. *high* resistance in one direction, low resistance in the other
    C. *high* resistance in both directions
    D. zero in both directions

19. The property of a coil which opposes current changes is called   19.___

    A. inductance   B. capacitance
    C. resistance   D. conductance

20. A push-pull circuit is used to   20.___

    A. double the frequency range that can be handled
    B. increase the harmonic content
    C. cancel out even harmonics, reduce hum, and increase power output
    D. increase total harmonic content and increase power output

21. A limiter tube in a FM receiver is operated

    A. with the plate at zero B+
    B. without a screen by-pass capacitor
    C. with low plate and screen voltages
    D. with large cathode resistors

22. The current flowing in the emitter circuit of a transistor consists of _____ current.

    A. collector
    B. base
    C. base and collector
    D. collector minus the base

23. Two 100 ohm, 10 watt resistors are connected in parallel. The net resistance and power rating will be _____ ohms at _____ watts.

    A. 200; 5
    B. 50; 10
    C. 100; 20
    D. 50; 20

24. If the emitter-base forward bias of a transistor *increases*, the

    A. emitter current remains constant
    B. collector current decreases
    C. base current approaches cutoff
    D. emitter current increases

25. The terminals of a junction FET are known as the

    A. emitter, base, and collector
    B. anode, cathode, and gate
    C. grid, cathode, and plate
    D. source, drain, and gate

KEY (CORRECT ANSWERS)

1.	B	11.	C
2.	C	12.	B
3.	C	13.	C
4.	B	14.	C
5.	D	15.	D
6.	C	16.	B
7.	B	17.	D
8.	B	18.	B
9.	A	19.	A
10.	A	20.	C

21. C
22. C
23. D
24. D
25. D

TEST 3

DIRECTIONS: Select the lettered word or phrase in Column II that matches the numbered item in Column I. Write the letter next to the corresponding number at the right.

COLUMN I

1. Inductance
2. Parallel
3. Zener diode
4. Reactance
5. Surge
6. Kilo
7. Farad
8. Source
9. Series
10. Attenuate
11. Cathode
12. Capacitor
13. Binary
14. Ampere
15. Current
16. Potentiometer
17. EMF
18. Anode
19. Amplification
20. Dielectric

COLUMN II

A. Unit of measure of current
B. Device that stores electrons
C. Electron flow
D. Insulator
E. Unit of measure of capacitors
F. Coil
G. Variable resistor with 3 contacts
H. Circuit with multiple paths
J. Regulated voltage supply
K. Device that supplies electrical power
L. Voltage
M. Metric prefix meaning one thousand
N. Increasing the strength of a signal
O. Positively charged electrode toward which electrons flow
P. To increase in strength
R. Number of systems using zeros and ones
S. Opposition to AC by a coil or capacitor
T. Element that emits electrons
U. Circuit in which current has one path
V. Sudden increase in voltage or current
W. Unit of measure of inductance
X. In series
Y. Provides protection in case of arcing
Z. Oscillator

1. _____
2. _____
3. _____
4. _____
5. _____
6. _____
7. _____
8. _____
9. _____
10. _____
11. _____
12. _____
13. _____
14. _____
15. _____
16. _____
17. _____
18. _____
19. _____
20. _____

KEY (CORRECT ANSWERS)

1.	F	11.	T
2.	H	12.	B
3.	J	13.	R
4.	S	14.	A
5.	V	15.	C
6.	M	16.	G
7.	E	17.	L
8.	K	18.	O
9.	U	19.	N
10.	P	20.	D

EXAMINATION SECTION
TEST 1

DIRECTIONS: Each question or incomplete statement is followed by several suggested answers or completions. Select the one that BEST answers the question or completes the statement. *PRINT THE LETTER OF THE CORRECT ANSWER IN THE SPACE AT THE RIGHT.*

1. The HIGHEST capacity among different condensers of the same size will be found in _____ condensers.

    A. mica
    B. paper
    C. electrolytic
    D. air

    1._____

2. To avoid shock hazard in handling the repair and testing of radio receivers, it is BEST to

    A. use an isolation transformer between the set and power outlet
    B. check all tubes first
    C. keep the chassis in the cabinet
    D. use a fused outlet

    2._____

3. Proper *dressing of leads* refers to the procedure involving

    A. reduction of soldered joints
    B. replacement of broken wires
    C. positioning of circuit wiring
    D. tightening of all contacts

    3._____

4. The MOST useful instrument in radio servicing is the

    A. vacuum tube voltmeter
    B. Wheatstone's bridge
    C. oscilloscope
    D. galvanometer

    4._____

5. Applying the raw rectified current to the plates of the vacuum tubes in an amplifier will cause

    A. distortion
    B. motor boating
    C. hum
    D. crackling

    5._____

6. Radio waves are

    A. electrostatic
    B. thermionic
    C. electrodynamic
    D. electromagnetic

    6._____

7. The presence of *snow* in a TV image is MOST commonly due to

    A. moist atmospheric conditions
    B. weak signal reception
    C. aging of the TV picture tube
    D. lack of suitable ground connection

    7._____

8. Shielding is often made use of in radio receivers as a means of

    A. increasing volume
    B. reducing gain
    C. decreasing power consumption
    D. reducing hum

    8._____

9. The PREFERRED soldering flux used in cleaning a joint to be soldered is a radio set is   9.____

    A. nitric acid   B. sal ammoniac
    C. rosin   D. casein

10. Miniaturization of transmitters and receivers has been accelerated by the employment of   10.____

    A. higher voltage sources   B. printed circuits
    C. electrostatic speakers   D. more efficient antennas

KEY (CORRECT ANSWERS)

1.	C	6.	D
2.	A	7.	B
3.	C	8.	D
4.	A	9.	C
5.	C	10.	B

TEST 2

DIRECTIONS: Each question or incomplete statement is followed by several suggested answers or completions. Select the one that BEST answers the question or completes the statement. *PRINT THE LETTER OF THE CORRECT ANSWER IN THE SPACE AT THE RIGHT.*

1. Misalignment of a TRF receiver is USUALLY caused by

    A. resistance
    B. conductance
    C. inductance
    D. capacity

2. A discussion about *woofer-tweeter* components would refer to

    A. high fidelity reproducers
    B. *walky-talky* devices
    C. radar installations
    D. transistor applications

3. The principle underlying the FM system of radio transmission and reception was originated by

    A. De Forest
    B. Armstrong
    C. Hartley
    D. Marconi

4. During a visit to the radio shop, a foreman observes a trainee wiping the tip of a hot soldering iron with a rag.
   This trainee should be

    A. told that the proper method is to shake the iron
    B. complimented
    C. told that the proper method is to dip the iron quickly into water
    D. told that the proper method is to permit the excess solder to drip off the tip

5. A requisition for switches for use of trainees in the construction of radios in the shop will contain relatively few classed as

    A. knife   B. toggle   C. rotary   D. slide

6. When checking the inventory of a beginner's radio shop, one would expect to find comparatively few

    A. potentiometers
    B. D.C. milliammeters
    C. capacitors
    D. oscillographs

7. *Ghosts* in television reception are MOST frequently caused by

    A. reflection of waves from nearby buildings
    B. incorrect antenna angle
    C. faulty vertical tube
    D. faulty horizontal tube

8. The type of radio receiver whose basic principle is the changing of the frequencies of all incoming stations to a single frequency is the

    A. T.R.F.
    B. super-heterodyne
    C. crystal
    D. neutradyne

9. Of the materials used in radio condensers, the one whose dielectric constant has the LOWEST value is 9.____

   A. air
   B. mica
   C. titanium dioxide
   D. paper

10. In the radio shop, holes in the metal chassis for tube bases are MOST commonly made with a 10.____

    A. coping saw
    B. center punch
    C. socket punch
    D. hacksaw

KEY (CORRECT ANSWERS)

1.	D	6.	D
2.	A	7.	B
3.	B	8.	B
4.	B	9.	A
5.	A	10.	C

EXAMINATION SECTION
TEST 1

DIRECTIONS: Answer the following questions directly, briefly, and succintly.

1. Why is the reactance of a series-tuned circuit zero at the resonant frequency?

2. What is the MOST important characteristic of a series-tuned circuit?

3. Under what circumstances will the voltage appearing across either the inductor or the capacitor in a series circuit be much higher than the source voltage?

4. Why is the impedance offered by a parallel-resonant circuit maximum and purely resistive at the resonant frequency?

5. Under what circumstances will an inductor and capacitor be in resonance at the same frequency irrespective of whether they are connected in series or in parallel?

6. What are two of the PRINCIPAL functions of tuned circuits in receivers?

7. What distinguishes a vector quantity from a sealer quantity?

8. How many times must the $+j$ operator be applied as a multiplying factor to a vector initially in the $0°$ position to rotate it $450°$?

9. If a vector. initially at the $0°$ position (along the $+X$ axis), is multiplied by j^3 and then by $-j^4$, what will be its angular position with respect to the X axis?

10. What magnitude and angle are represented by the expression $j^2 5$?

SOLUTIONS TO PROBLEMS

1. Because X_L and X_C are equal and opposite in polarity and therefore cancel each other.

2. The circuit impedance is a minimum at resonance, thereby allowing maximum current flow.

3. At a resonance, when the effective series resistance is low.

4. Because the currents in the two branches are approximately 180° out of phase and combine to produce a small resultant.

5. When the ratio of reactance to the inherent resistance in each unit is high.

6. To select the desired frequencies and to reject the undesired frequencies.

7. A vector quantity has magnitude and direction; a scalar quantity has only magnitude.

8. 5 times.

9. 90° clockwise from the 0° position, or -90°.

10. 5 units long and 180°.

TEST 2

DIRECTIONS: Answer the following questions directly, briefly, and succinctly.

1. What are the three PRINCIPAL uses of electron tubes?
2. In thermionic emission, what causes the electrons to gain enough energy to escape from the emitter?
3. In photoelectric emission, what determines the velocity of the emitted electrons?
4. What is the PRINCIPAL advantage of tungsten emitters?
5. In what classes of tubes are thoriated-tungsten emitters used?
6. What type of emitter is used in MOST types of receiving tubes?
7. Why are indirectly heated cathodes seldom used in portable equipment?
8. Why are electron tubes generally evacuated?
9. In electron-tube operation what is the meaning of the term *saturation voltage*?
10. At low values of plate voltage, how is plate current controlled?

2 (#2)

SOLUTIONS TO PROBLEMS

1. To convert currents and voltages from one waveform to another, to amplify weak signals, and to generate high-frequency currents.

2. Heat

3. The frequency of the incident radiant energy.

4. Their great durability.

5. Medium power tubes with plate voltage between 500 and 5,000 volts.

6. Oxide-coated emitter.

7. Too much power is required for heating purposes.

8. To prevent oxidation of the cathode and heating element and to permit the flow of current from cathode to plate without colliding with gas particles.

9. The plate voltage at which all of the electrons transmitted by the cathode are attracted to the plate.

10. By the voltage between plate and cathode.

TEST 3

DIRECTIONS: Answer the following questions directly, briefly, and succinctly.

1. How does the B-supply differ from the A-supply?

2. Why is it important in a directly heated cathode to return the grid and plate circuits of a tube to a point the exact electrical center of the filament circuit when a.c. is used for heating?

3. Why is the center-tap grid and plate return not needed when indirectly heated cathodes are used?

4. What type of rectifier tube (high-vacuum or gas-filled) is MOST widely used in low-current applications?

5. What are two of the important characteristics of the high-vacuum rectifier tube?

6. Why is the mercury-vapor rectifier MORE efficient than the high-vacuum rectifier?

7. What is the normal voltage drop across a mercury rectifiers tube when it is conducting?

8. Why is the peak inverse voltage rating of the individual copper-oxide rectifier units relatively low?

9. How may the peak inverse voltage rating of dry-disk rectifier be increased?

10. What are the rms and average values of the unfiltered voltage across a load supplied by a full-wave rectifier having a peak output voltage of 200 volts?

SOLUTIONS TO PROBLEMS

1. The B-supply is always d.c. and supplies high-voltage at low current; the A-supply may supply either a.c. or d.c. and furnishes low voltage at relatively high current.

2. To minimize hum caused by the a.c. heater component modulating the space current.

3. The heating and emitting elements are electrically insulated and therefore the a.c. heater component is not coupled to the signal circuits.

4. High-vacuum tube.

5. Maximun peak plate current and maximum inverse peak plate voltage rating.

6. Because of the lower voltage drop across the mercury-vapor tube resulting in less power loss in the tube.

7. 15 volts.

8. The oxide coating is thin and therefore may be easily punctured.

9. By connecting a number of units in series.

10. 141.4 volts and 127.2 volts respectively.

TEST 4

DIRECTIONS: Answer the following questions directly, briefly, and succinctly.

1. Which component (a.c or d.c) of the voltages and current in an amplifier circuit determines the portion of the tube characteristic at which operation occurs?
2. How may transformer coupling make the gain of a stage greater or less than mu?
3. What is the PRIMARY function of voltage amplifiers?
4. Express the formula for the gain of a voltage amplifier in terms of the output and input voltages.
5. Define power amplification.
6. Define plate efficiency.
7. Define power sensitivity.
8. During what part of the input cycle does plate current flow in a class-A amplifier?
9. What is the action of class-B audio amplifiers connected in push-pull?
10. During what part of the input cycle does plate current flow in a class-AB amplifier?

SOLUTIONS TO PROBLEMS

1. The d.c. component.

2. By having a step-up or a step-down turns ratio.

3. To increase the relatively low amplitude of an input signal on the grid to a relatively high amplitude in the output (plate) circuit.

4. Voltage gain = $\dfrac{\text{signal voltage output}}{\text{signal voltage input}}$

5. The ratio of the output power to the input grid driving power.

6. The ratio of useful output power to d.c. input power in the plate circuit.

7. The ratio of the output power in watts to the square of the effective value of grid signal voltage.

8. The entire cycle.

9. Each tube supplies that half of the waveform not supplied by the other, thus giving a true reproduction of the input signal.

10. It flows for more than half but less than the full cycle.

TEST 5

DIRECTIONS: Answer the following questions directly, briefly, and succinctly.

1. Name (a) three types of electromechanical loads and
    (b) two control functions that are applicable to d.c. amplifier outputs.

2. What is the effect of positive feedback on amplifier gain and selectivity.

3. What is the effect of positive feedback on undesirable distortion introduced within the amplifier itself?

4. What is the effect of negative feedback on nonlinear distortion in an amplifier stage?

5. Why cannot distortion that is introduced in the first stage of an amplifier be eliminated by negative feedback applied across the last stage?

6. In which amplifier stages (high- or low-level) is feedback more effective?

7. If the high frequencies are to be amplified more than the low frequencies, what frequencies must be attenuated in the feedback network?

8. How does negative feedback affect the gain of an amplifier?

9. Negative feedback employing current feedback may be simply accomplished by leaving out which of the circuit elements?

10. What are the relative values of circuit Q and g_m in a high-gain single-tuned transformer-coupled amplifier?

SOLUTIONS TO PROBLEMS

11. a. Meter, relay and counter:
    b. gain control of an amplifier, and frequency control of an oscillator.

12. Both gain and selectivity are increased.

13. The undesirable distortion is increased.

14. The nonlinear distortion is reduced.

15. Because it must occur in the plate circuit of the stage across which feedback is to be applied in order to separate the distortion from the desired signal.

16. In the high-level stages.

17. The high frequencies.

18. The gain is reduced.

19. The cathode resistor bypass capacitor.

20. They are both high.

EXAMINATION SECTION
TEST 1

DIRECTIONS: Answer the following questions directly, briefly and succinctly.

1. What is the PRIMARY function of a power amplifier?   1._____

2. Give three general characteristics of audio power amplifiers.   2._____

3. In a class-A power amplifier, what characteristics of the i_p-e_g curve limits the minimum value of i_p?   3._____

4. For MAXIMUM undistorted power output in a class-A triode power amplifier, what is the relative value of load impedance with respect to the plate resistance of the triode?   4._____

5. Why is the efficiency of a class-A amplifier low?   5._____

6. State the equation of the load line for a power amplifier in terms of the plate current, plate load resistance, and plate supply voltage.   6._____

7. If the maximum value of the second harmonic current is 0.8 ma and the maximum value of the fundamental is 20 ma, what is the percentage of distortion due to the second harmonic?   7._____

8. Express the equation of the primary-to-secondary turns ratio of a transformer in terms of the primary-to-secondary matching impedances.   8._____

9. What causes the reduced high-frequency response of an output transformer?   9._____

10. What characteristics must an output transformer have to extend the flat portion of the frequency-response curve of the output transformer into both the low- and the high-frequency regions?   10._____

SOLUTIONS TO PROBLEMS

1. To deliver power to a load.

2. Low amplification factors, low plate resistance, and high plate current.

3. The curvature of the lower portion of the curve.

4. The load impedance is twice the plate resistance.

5. Because appreciable plate current flows during the entire grid-voltage cycle.

6. $e_p = E_b - i_p R_L$.

7. 4 percent.

8. The primary-to-secondary turns ratio is equal to the square root of the primary-to-secondary matching impedances.

9. The loss in voltage through the transformer primary and secondary leakage reactance as a result of (1) load current and (2) capacitative current due to shunting capacitance.

10. High primary inductance and low leakage inductance.

TEST 2

DIRECTIONS: Answer the following questions directly, briefly and succinctly.

1. What are two conditions necessary to produce sustained oscillations in an electron-tube oscillator?   1._____

2. What determines the upper frequency limit of electron-tube oscillators?   2._____

3. In a tickler-feedback oscillator what grid circuit test may be made to indicate proper operation?   3._____

4. In a series-fed Hartley oscillator what action maintains the oscillations in the tank circuit when the plate current is zero and no energy is being supplied to the oscillator circuit?   4._____

5. What is the advantage of self-bias in a series-fed Hartley oscillator?   5._____

6. What circuit arrangement distinguishes the shunt-fed Hartley oscillator from the series-fed type?   6._____

7. How does the voltage divider in the Colpitts oscillator tank circuit differ from the one used In the Hartley oscillator?   7._____

8. How is feedback obtained in a tuned-plate tuned-grid oscillator?   8._____

9. Which tuned circuti in terms of the relative tank circuit Q (high or low) in a TPTG oscillator determines the oscillator frequency?   9._____

10. Push-pull oscillators are generally used in what frequency ranges?   10._____

SOLUTIONS TO PROBLEMS

1. The feedback must be regenerative, and the feedback energy must be sufficient to compensate for the energy losses in the grid circuit.

2. The distributed inductance and capacitance of the circuit components and the interelectrode capacitance of the tubes.

3. Measurement of the d.c. voltage developed across the grid resistor.

4. The flywheel, effect (interchange of energy between the tank coil and capacitor).

5. It makes the oscillator self-starting.

6. The d.c. component of plate current is isolated from the tuned circuit in the shunt-fed Hartley oscillator.

7. The Colpitts oscillator uses a split-tank capacitor instead of a split-tank inductor.

8. Through the plate-grid interelectrode capacitance of the tube.

9. The circuit having the higher Q.

10. In the high- and ultrahigh-frequency ranges.

TEST 3

DIRECTIONS: Answer the following questions directly, briefly and succinctly.

1. In what frequency components of the a-m wave is the intelligence contained? 1.____
2. What percentage of modulation corresponds to the condition of MAXIMUM permissible power in the side bands? 2.____
3. Why is the band of frequencies that may be transmitted on a-m restricted? 3.____
4. For 100-percent modulation, what relation exists between the af and r-f input power? 4.____
5. When 100percent modulation occurs, what is the percentage increase in antenna current over the unmodulated value? 5.____
6. What is the relative magnitude of the peak power output of the transmitter r-f amplifier during 100-percent modulation compared with that of the unmodulated peak power output? 6.____
7. What class of r-f amplifier is USUALLY used with high-level plate modulation for maximum efficiency and ease of adjustment? 7.____
8. What are the advantages of grid modulation? 8.____
9. What are the disadvantages of grid modulation? 9.____
10. Why may a tone-modulated carrier be modulated approximately 100-percent? 10.____

SOLUTIONS TO PROBLEMS

1. In the side bands.

2. 100 percent.

3. To prevent interference with other channels.

4. The a-f input is equal to one-half the r-f input.

5. 22.4 percent

6. It is four times as great.

7. Class C.

8. Space, weight, and input power are less than for plate modulation.

9. The degree of modulation, the power, and the intelligibility are reduced.

10. Because a buzzer or audio oscillator having a constant amplitude output voltage is used as the tone source.

TEST 4

DIRECTIONS: Answer the following questions directly, briefly and succinctly.

1. For a given transmitter, why does cw have a GEEATER range than mcw or voice modulation? 1.____

2. Why is the very-low frequency band NOT covered by shipboard transmitters? 2.____

3. What is an advantage of using the very-low-frequency band? 3.____

4. Which frequency band is used for radar? 4.____

5. What is a disadvantage of using crystal-controlled oscillators in transmitters operating at the lower frequencies? 5.____

6. How is frequency drift eliminated in transmitters? 6.____

7. What type of oscillator is COMMONLY used in the lower frequency ranges? 7.____

8. Why are frequency multipliers COMMONLY used with crystal controlled oscillators? 8.____

9. How does the output of a frequency multiplier vary with the extent of frequency multiplication? 9.____

10. What three important conditions MUST prevail in; an amplifier in order to obtain frequency multiplication? 10.____

SOLUTIONS TO PROBLEMS

1. Because c-w has fewer side bands and therefore greater signal strength in the remaining side-band frequencies.

2. Because the antennas are too long.

3. The signals are capable of being transmitted through magnetic storms that blank out the higher r-f channels.

4. The upper end of the ultrahigh-frequency band.

5. The large number of crystals needed.

6. By placing the frequency-determining components of the oscillator in a temperature-controlled oven, loading the oscillator very lightly, and isolating it with a. buffer stage.

7. The electron-coupled oscillator (ECO).

8. So that the crystal may be operated at a lower frequency and therefore be larger and more rugged.

9. Inversely.

10. (1) High-grid driving voltage, (2) high grid bias, and (3) the plate tank tuned to the desired harmonic.

TEST 5

DIRECTIONS: Answer the following questions directly, briefly and succinctly.

1. What are four uses of resonant r-f lines other than for the transmission of power? 1.____

2. What is the effect on the characteristic impedance of a two-wire line if the wires are moved farther apart? 2.____

3. What is the phase relation between voltage and current on a line of infinite length? 3.____

4. Why do the waveforms diminish in amplitude along a line of infinite length? 4.____

5. What is the constant ratio of voltage to current called on a line that is terminated in an impedance equal to this ratio? 5.____

6. What is the relative magnitude of the load impedance compared with the characteristic impedance of a nonresonant line? 6.____

7. In an open-end resonant line, why is the impedance prevented from being zero at odd quarter-wavelengths from the terminal end of the line? 7.____

8. What type of circuit would a generator "see" if it is connected one-half wavelength from the end of an open-end resonant line? 8.____

9. What type of circuit would a generator "see" if it is connected three-eighths wavelength from the end of an open-end resonant line? 9.____

10. A shorted transmission line one-half wavelength long acts like what kind of circuit? 10.____

SOLUTIONS TO PROBLEMS

1. They may be used as (1) impedance-matching devices, (2) phase shifters and inverters, (3) wave filters and chokes, and (4) oscillator frequency controls.

2. The characteristic impedance is increased.

3. They are in phase.

4. Because of line losses.

5. The characteristic impedance.

6. They are equal.

7. Because of circuit losses.

8. A parallel-resonant circuit having high resistance.

9. An inductor.

10. A series resonant circuit.

EXAMINATION SECTION
TEST 1

DIRECTIONS: Answer the following questions directly, briefly, and succinctly.

1. State a basic principle of the radiation of electromagnetic energy that pertains to a moving electric field and its associated magnetic component; also to a moving magnetic field and its associated electric field component.

2. State the formula for the wavelength of an electromagnetic wave in free space in terms of the frequency of the radiating source and the speed of the wave. (Assume the wavelength is in meters and the frequency is in megacycles.)

3. If the r-f generator supplying a tuned dipole antenna has a voltage output of sine waveform, what is the waveform of the antenna current distribution with respect to the length of the dipole?

4. At what approximate distance in wavelengths from an antenna does the induction field become negligible?

5. How does the strength of the radiated field vary with distance?

6. Why are resonant conductors more efficient radiators than non-resonant conductors?

7. What is the relative velocity of the radio wave in an antenna compared to that of the wave in free space?

8. What determines the magnitude of the antenna current at the feedpoint for a given r-f voltage at that point?

9. Why is a large-diameter radiator physically shorter than a small-diameter radiator, assuming the same resonant frequency in both cases?

10. Define radiation resistance.

KEY (CORRECT ANSWERS)

1. A moving electric field creates a magnetic field and a moving magnetic field creates an electric field.

2. $\lambda = \dfrac{300}{f}$

3. Sine waveform

4. At few wavelengths

5. Inversely

6. Because they have large standing waves of voltage and current with a minimum of generator current and voltage

7. Less

8. The antenna input impedance

9. Because the large-diameter radiator has greater capacitance hence less inductance

10. Radiation resistance is the value of resistance that will dissipate the same power that the antenna dissipates.

TEST 2

DIRECTIONS: Answer the following questions directly, briefly, and succinctly.

1. Distinguish between selectivity and sensitivity of a receiver.

2. What are two reasons tetrodes or pentodes are generally used in r-f amplifiers?

3. When a common B supply is used in a multistage amplifier why does the greatest amount of feedback occur between the final and first amplifier stages?

4. What are R-C circuits called that are designed specifically to counteract feedback in both r-f and a-f amplifiers?

5. What is the function of so-called electrical or mechanical bandspread used in receiver tuning?

6. What are two functions of an a-m detector?

7. What portion of the i_p-e_g curve, on which the plate detector is operated, accounts for the introduction of some distortion?

8. In most cases, what determines the amount of amplification required in the a-f section of a receiver?

9. What is the relative magnitude of the secondary impedance compared with that of the voice coil?

10. In a permanent-magnet dynamic type of loudspeaker, to what electrical quantity is the force on the voice coil proportional?

2 (#2)

KEY (CORRECT ANSWERS)

1. Selectivity is the ability to select the desired signal; sensitivity is the ability to amplify weak signals.

2. Because, unlike triodes, they usually do not require neutralization, and they have higher gain.

3. Because of the high amplification through the multistage amplifier.

4. Decoupling circuits

5. To separate stations that are crowded together on the dial

6. (1) To rectify the signal, and
   (2) to filter it (remove the r-f component and pass the a-f component on to the a-f amplifier)

7. The curved portion near the cutoff point

8. The type of reproducer

9. They are equal

10. To the a-c signal current in the voice coil

TEST 3

DIRECTIONS: Answer the following questions directly, briefly, and succinctly.

1. What is the primary function of the cathode-ray oscilloscope as a test instrument?

2. How does the operator of a cathode-ray oscilloscope determine whether the pattern of a waveform is correct for the circuit under test?

3. What are the two types of deflection used in cathode-ray tubes?

4. In what type of deflection is the field that causes the deflection produced outside the cathode-ray tube?

5. In a cathode-ray tube, what controls the electron beam intensity?

6. What is the purpose of the second anode in a cathode-ray tube?

7. Why are the cathode-ray beam electrons not mutually repelled enough to defocus the beam?

8. How is focusing in an electrostatic-type cathode-ray tube generally controlled?

9. After the focus coil in an electromagnetic cathode-ray tube has been properly positioned, how is focusing accomplished?

10. What is meant by the electron beam deflection angle in a cathode-ray tube?

2 (#3)

KEY (CORRECT ANSWERS)

1. To produce a visual presentation of circuit waveforms

2. By comparing the observed waveforms with the optimum efficiency waveforms printed on the schematic diagrams or on the equipment

3. Electrostatic and electromagnetic

4. Electromagnetic deflection

5. A cylindrical grid surrounding the cathode

6. To accelerate the electrons in the beam and aid in the focus action

7. Because of their high velocity in the direction of the screen

8. By varying the voltage between the first anode and the cathode

9. By varying the current through the focus coil

10. The angle through which the beam may be deflected in any direction from the center line through the tube

TEST 4

DIRECTIONS: Answer the following questions directly, briefly, and succinctly.

1. If a person shouts in the direction of a cliff and there is a 2-second interval before he hears the echo, how far is the cliff? (Assume the velocity of sound in air to be 1,100 ft/sec.)

2. What effect is utilized in the continuous-wave radar method of detecting a target?

3. In the frequency-modulation radar method, upon what does the frequency difference of the outgoing and incoming signals depend?

4. Why are the problems experienced with the c-w and f-m radar methods not present in pulse radar?

5. What are the three general classifications of radar equipment?

6. What type of information is given in type-A presentation?

7. What type of information is given in type-B and PPI presentation?

8. How far (in yards) do radio waves travel in 1 microsecond?

9. How long (in microseconds) does it take a radio wave to travel 1 nautical mile (2,000 yards)?

10. What is the relation between the time for one sweep on the radar screen and the time for the transmitted pulse to travel to the target (maximum range) and return to the receiver?

2 (#4)

KEY (CORRECT ANSWERS)

1. 1,100 feet

2. Doppler effect

3. The distance traveled by the signals

4. Pulse radar does not depend on the relative frequency of the returned signal or on the motion of the target.

5. Search, fire control, and fighter-director

6. Range

7. Range and azimuth angle

8. 328 yards

9. 6.1 microseconds

10. The time is the same in both cases.

TEST 5

DIRECTIONS: Answer the following questions directly, briefly, and succinctly.

1. What is the effect on the accuracy of a radar of making the antenna beam angle narrower?

2. How may the altitude of a target be determined if the slant range and the angle of elevation are known?

3. What type of presentation has a radial time-base line?

4. How is the radar echo applied to the (1) range scope and (2) PPI scope?

5. In order to locate targets at long range, search radars have what special design features?

6. In order to obtain precision target resolution at short range, fire control radars have what special design features?

7. What are the functions of the timer, or keyer, in a radar system?

8. What is the function of the transmitter in a radar system?

9. What is the relation between carrier frequency and the size of the radar antenna array for a given sharpness of pattern?

10. What is one of the problems involved when the size of an electron tube is reduced in order to reduce interelectrode capacitances and transit time?

KEY (CORRECT ANSWERS)

1. The accuracy is increased.

2. The altitude is equal to the slant range multiplied by the sine of the angle of elevation.

3. PPI

4. (1) In the range scope it is amplified and applied to the vertical deflection plate in such a way as to produce a pip on the horizontal time base line on the screen;
   (2) In the PPI scope it is amplified and applied to the control grid in such a way that the trace is brightened momentarily on the radial time base line on the screen.

5. High power, wide beam angle, and long pulse widths

6. Relatively low power, short pulse width, and narrow beam angle

7. It produces the synchronizing signals that trigger the transmitter; triggers the indicator sweep; and coordinates the other associated circuits.

8. To generate r-f energy in short, powerful pulses

9. The higher the carrier frequency, the smaller is the antenna array.

10. The power rating is reduced.

GLOSSARY OF ELECTRONIC TERMS

TABLE OF CONTENTS

	Page
Acorn Tube … Bias	1
Biasing Resistor … Coefficient of Coupling (K)	2
Condenser … Dielectric	3
Dielectric Constant … Electrostatic Field	4
Equivalent Circuit … Henry (h)	5
Helmholts Coil … Klystron	6
Lag … Neutralisation	7
Node … Plate Resistance (r_p)	8
Positive Feedback … Relaxation Oscillator	9
Reluctance … Solenoid	10
Space Charge … Unbalanced Line	11
Unidirectional … Z	12

ELECTRONICS SYMBOLS

Amplifier … Cell, Photosensitive	13
Circuit Breaker … Discontinuity	14
Electron Tube … Inductor	15
Key, Telegraph … Meter, Instrument	16
Mode Transducer … Semiconductor Device	17
Squib … Transformer	18
Vibrator, Interrupter … Visual Signaling Device	19

TRANSISTOR SYMBOLS — 19

TUBE SYMBOLS — 20

GLOSSARY OF ELECTRONIC TERMS

Acorn tube. An acorn-shaped vacuum tube designed for ultra-high-frequency circuits. The tube has short electron transit time and low inter-electrode capacitance because of close spacing and small size electrodes.

Align. To adjust the tuned circuits of a receiver or transmitter for maximum signal response.

Alternation. One-half of a complete cycle.

Ammeter. An instrument for measuring the electron flow in amperes.

Ampere (amp). The basic unit of current or electron flow.

Amplification (A). The process of increasing the strength of a signal.

Amplification factor (ft). The ratio of a small change in plate voltage to a small change in grid voltage, with all other electrode voltages constant, required to produce the same small change in plate current.

Amplifier. A device used to increase the signal voltage, current, or power, generally composed of a vacuum tube and associated circuit called a stage. It may contain several stages in order to obtain a desired gain.

Amplitude. The maximum instantaneous value of an alternating voltage or current, measured in either the positive or negative direction.

Amplitude distortion. The changing of a waveshape so that it is no longer proportional to its original form. Also known as harmonic distortion.

Anode. A positive electrode; the plate of a vacuum tube.

Antenna. A device used to radiate or absorb r-f energy.

Aquadag. A graphite coating on the inside of certain cathode-ray tubes for collecting secondary electrons emitted by the screen.

Array (antenna). An arrangement of antenna elements, usually di-poles, which results in desirable directional characteristics.

Attenuation. The reduction in the strength of a signal.

Audio frequency (a-f). A frequency which can be detected as a sound by the human ear. The range of audio frequencies extends approximately from 20 to 20,000 cycles per second.

Autodyne circuit. A circuit in which the same elements and vacuum tube are used as an oscillator and as a detector. The output has a frequency equal to the difference between the frequencies of the received signal and the oscillator signal.

Automatic gain control (age) A method of automatically regulating the gain of a receiver so that the output tends to remain constant though the incoming signal may vary in strength.

Automatic volume control (avc). See Automatic gain control.

Autotransformer. A transformer in which part of the primary winding is used as a secondary winding, or vice versa.

Azimuth. The angular measurement in a horizontal plane and in a clockwise direction, beginning at a point oriented to north.

Ballast resistance. A self-regulating resistance, usually connected in the primary circuit of a power transformer to compensate for variations in the line voltage.

Ballast tube. A tube which contains a ballast resistance.

Band of frequencies. The frequencies existing between two definite limits.

Band-pass filter. A circuit designed to pass with nearly equal response all currents having frequencies within a definite band, and to reduce substantially the amplitudes of currents of all frequencies outside that band.

Bazooka. See Line-balance converter.

Beam-power tube. A high vacuum tube in which the electron stream is directed in concentrated beams from the cathode to the plate. Variously termed beam-power tetrode and beam-power pentode.

Beat frequency. A frequency resulting from the combination of two different frequencies. It is numerically equal to the difference between or the sum of these two frequencies.

Beat note. See Beat frequency.

Bias. The average d-c voltage maintained between the cathode and control grid of a vacuum tube.

Biasing resistor. A resistor used to provide the voltage drop for a required bias.

Blanking. See Gating.

Bleeder. A resistance connected in parallel with a power-supply output to protect equipment from excessive voltages if the load is removed or substantially reduced; to improve the voltage regulation, and to drain the charge remaining in the filter capacitors when the unit is turned off.

Blocking capacitor. A capacitor used to block the flow of direct current while permitting the flow of alternating current.

Break-down voltage. The voltage at which an insulator or dielectric ruptures, or at which ionization and conduction take place in a gas or vapor.

Brilliance modulation. See Intensity modulation.

Buffer amplifier. An amplifier used to isolate the output of an oscillator from the effects produced by changes in voltage or loading in following circuits.

Buncher. The electrode of a velocity-modulated tube which alters the velocity of electrons in the constant current beam causing the electrons to become bunched in a drift space beyond the buncher electrode.

Bypass capacitor. A capacitor used to provide an alternating current path of comparatively low impedance around a circuit element.

Capacitance. The property of two or more bodies which enables them to store electrical energy in an electrostatic field between the bodies.

Capacitive coupling. A method of transferring energy from one circuit to another by means of a capacitor that is common to both circuits.

Capacitive reactance (X_c). The opposition offered to the flow of an alternating current by capacitance, expressed in ohms.

Capacitor. Two electrodes or sets of electrodes in the form of plates, separated from each other by an insulating material called the dielectric.

Carrier. The r-f component of a transmitted wave upon which an audio signal or other form of intelligence can be impressed.

Catcher. The electrode of a velocity-modulated tube which receives energy from the bunched electrons.

Cathode (K). The electrode in a vacuum tube which is the source of electron emission. Also a negative electrode.

Cathode bias. The method of biasing a tube by placing the biasing resistor in the common cathode return circuit, making the cathode more positive, rather than the grid more negative, with respect to ground.

Cathode follower. A vacuum-tube circuit in which the input signal is applied between the control grid and ground, and the output is taken from the cathode and ground. A cathode follower has a high input impedance and a low output impedance.

Characteristic impedance (Z_0). The ratio of the voltage to the current at every point along a transmission line on which there are no standing waves.

Choke. A coil which impedes the flow of alternating current of a specified frequency range because of its high inductive reactance at that range.

Chopping. See Limiting.

Clamping circuit. A circuit which maintains either amplitude extreme of a waveform at a certain level of potential.

Class A operation. Operation of a vacuum tube so that plate current flows throughout the entire operating cycle and distortion is kept to a minimum.

Class AB operation. Operation of a vacuum tube with grid bias so that the operating point is approximately halfway between Class A and Class B.

Class B operation. Operation of a vacuum tube with bias at or near cut-off so that plate current flows during approximately one-half cycle.

Class C operation. Operation of a vacuum tube with bias considerably beyond cut-off so that plate current flows for less than one-half cycle.

Clipping. See Limiting.

Coaxial cable. A transmission line consisting of two conductors concentric with and insulated from each other.

Coefficient of coupling (K). A numerical indication of the degree of coupling existing between two circuits, expressed in terms of either a decimal or a percentage.

Condenser. See Capacitor.

Conductance (G). The ability of a material to conduct or carry an electric current. It is the reciprocal of the resistance of the material, and is expressed in *ohms.*

Continuous waves. Radio waves which maintain a constant amplitude and a constant frequency.

Control grid (G). The electrode of a vacuum tube other than a diode upon which the signal voltage is impressed in order to control the plate current.

Control-grid-plate transconductance. See Transconductance.

Conversion transconductance (gc). A characteristic associated with the mixer function of vacuum tubes, and used in the same manner as transconductance is used. It is the ratio of the i-f current in the primary of the first i-f transformer to the r-f signal voltage producing it.

Converter. See Mixer.

Converter tube. A multielement vacuum tube used both as a mixer and as an oscillator in a superheterodyne receiver. It creates a local frequency and combines it with an incoming signal to produce an intermediate frequency.

Counting circuit. A circuit which receives uniform pulses representing units to be counted and produces a voltage in proportion to their frequency.

Coupled impedance. The effect produced in the primary winding of a transformer by the influence of the current flowing in the secondary winding.

Coupling. The association of two circuits in such a way that energy may be transferred from one to the other.

Coupling element. The means by which energy is transferred from one circuit to another; the common impedance necessary for coupling.

Critical coupling. The degree of coupling which provides the maximum transfer of energy between two resonant circuits at the resonant frequency.

Crystal (Xtal). (1) A natural substance, such as quartz or tourmaline, which is capable of producing a voltage stress when under pressure, or producing pressure when under an applied voltage. Under stress it has the property of responding only to a given frequency when cut to a given thickness.

(2) A nonlinear element such as gelena or silicon, in which case the piezo-electric characteristic is not exhibited.

Crystal mixer. A device which employs the nonlinear characteristic of a crystal (nonpiezo-electric type) and a point contact to mix two frequencies.

Crystal oscillator. An oscillator circuit in which a piezoelectric crystal is used to control the frequency and to reduce frequency instability to a minimum.

Current (J). Flow of electrons; measured in amperes.

Cut-off (c.o.). The minimum value of negative grid bias which prevents the flow of plate current in a vacuum tube.

Cut-off limiting. Limiting the maximum output voltage of a vacuum-tube circuit by driving the grid beyond cut-off.

Cycle. One complete positive and one complete negative alternation of a current or voltage.

Damped waves. Waves which decrease exponentially in amplitude.

Decoupling network. A network of capacitors and chokes, or resistors, placed in leads which are common to two or more circuits to prevent unwanted interstage coupling.

Deflection sensitivity (CRT). The quotient of the displacement of the electron beam at the place of impact by the change in the deflecting field. It is usually expressed in millimeters per volt applied between the deflection electrodes, or in millimeters per gauss of the deflecting magnetic field.

Degeneration. The process whereby a part of the output signal of an amplifying device is returned to its input circuit in such a manner that it tends to cancel the input.

De-ionization potential. The potential at which ionization of the gas within a gas-filled tube ceases and conduction stops.

Demodulation. See Detection.

Detection. The process of separating the modulation component from the received signal.

Dielectric. An insulator; a term applied to the

insulating material between the plates of a capacitor.

Dielectric constant. The ratio of the capacitance of a capacitor with a dielectric between the electrodes to the capacitance with air between the electrodes.

Differentiating circuit. A circuit which produces an output voltage substantially in proportion to the rate of change of the input voltage.

Diode. A two-electrode vacuum tube containing a cathode and a plate.

Diode detector. A detector circuit employing a diode tube.

Dipole antenna. Two metallic elements, each approximately one quarter wavelength long, which radiate r-f energy fed to them by the transmission line.

Directly heated cathode. A filament cathode which carries its own heating current for electron emission, as distinguished from an indirectly heated cathode.

Director (antenna). A parasitic antenna placed in front of a radiating element so that r-f radiation is aided in the forward direction.

Distortion. The production of an output waveform which is not a true reproduction of the input waveform. Distortion may consist of irregularities in amplitude, frequency, or phase.

Distributed capacitance. The capacitance that exists between the turns in a coil or choke, or between adjacent conductors or circuits, as dis- tinguished from the capacitance which is concentrated in a capacitor.

Distributed inductance. The inductance that exists along the entire length of a conductor, as distinguished from the self-inductance which is concentrated in a coil.

Doorknob tube. A doorknob-shaped vacuum tube designed for ultra-high-frequency circuits. This tube has short electron transit time and low interelectrode capacitance, because of the close spacing and small size of electrodes.

Dropping resistor. A resistor used to decrease a given voltage to a lower value.

Dry electrolytic capacitor. An electrolytic capacitor using a paste instead of a liquid electrolyte. *See* Electrolytic capacitor.

Dynamic characteristics. The relation between the instantaneous plate voltage and plate current of a vacuum tube as the voltage applied to the grid is moved; thus, the characteristics of a vacuum tube during operation.

Dynatron. A negative resistance device; particularly, a tetrode operating on that portion of its i_p vs. e_p characteristic where secondary emission exists to such an extent that an increase in plate voltage actually causes a decrease in plate current, and, therefore, makes the circuit behave like a negative resistance.

Eccles-Jordan circuit (trigger circuit). A direct coupled multivibrator circuit possessing two conditions of stable equilibrium. Also known as a flip-flop circuit.

Effective value. The equivalent heating value of an alternating current or voltage, as compared to a direct current or voltage. It is 0.707 times the peak value of a sine wave. It is also called the rms value.

Efficiency. The ratio of output to input power, generally expressed as a percentage.

Electric field. A space in which an electric charge will experience a force exerted upon it.

Electrode. A terminal at which electricity passes from one medium into another.

Electrolyte. A water solution of a substance which is capable of conducting electricity. An electrolyte may be in the form of either a liquid or a paste.

Electrolytic capacitor. A capacitor employing a metallic plate and an electrolyte as the second plate separated by a dielectric which is produced by electrochemical action.

Electromagnetic field. A space field in which electric and magnetic vectors at right angles to each other travel in a direction at right angles to both.

Electron. The negatively charged particles of matter. The smallest particle of matter.

Electron emission. The liberation of electrons from a bo]difference.

Electronic switch. A circuit which causes a start-and-stop action or a switching action by electronic means.

Electronic voltmeter. *See* Vacuum tube voltmeter.

Electrostatic field. The field of influence

between two charged bodies.

Equivalent circuit. A diagrammatic arrangement of coils, resistors, and capacitors, representing the effects of a more complicated circuit in order to permit easier analysis.

Farad (f). The unit of capacitance.

Feedback. A transfer of energy from the output circuit of a device back to its input.

Field. The space containing electric or magnetic lines of force.

Field intensity. Electrical strength of a field.

Filament. See Directly heated cathode.

Filter. A combination of circuit elements designed to pass a definite range of frequencies, attenuating all others.

Firing potential. The controlled potential at which conduction through a gas-filled tube begins.

First detector. See Mixer.

Fixed bias. A bias voltage of constant value, such as one obtained from a battery, power supply, or generator.

Fixed capacitor. A capacitor which has no provision for varying its capacitance.

Fixed resistor. A resistor which has no provision for varying its resistance.

Fluorescence. The property of emitting light as the immediate result of electronic bombardment.

Fly-back. The portion of the time base during which the spot is returning to the starting point. This is usually not seen on the screen of the cathode-ray tube, because of gating action or the rapidity with which it occurs.

Free electrons. Electrons which are loosely held and consequently tend to move at random among the atoms of the material.

Free oscillations. Oscillatory currents which continue to flow in a tuned circuit after the impressed voltage has been removed. Their frequency is the resonant frequency of the tuned circuit.

Frequency (f). The number of complete cycles per second existing in any form of wave motion; such as the number of cycles per second of an alternating current.

Frequency distortion. Distortion which occurs as a result of failure to amplify or attenuate equally all frequencies present in a complex wave.

Frequency modulation. See Modulation.

Frequency stability. The ability of an oscillator to maintain its operation at a constant frequency.

Full-wave rectifier circuit. A circuit which utilizes both the positive and the negative alternations of an alternating current to produce a direct current.

Gain (A). The ratio of the output power, voltage, or current to the input power, voltage, or current, respectively.

Gas tube. A tube filled with gas at low pressure in order to obtain certain desirable characteristics.

Gating (cathode-ray tube). Applying a rectangular voltage to the grid or cathode of a cathode-ray tube to sensitize it during the sweep time only.

Grid current. Current which flows between the cathode and the grid whenever the grid becomes positive with respect to the cathode.

Grid detection. Detection by rectification in the grid circuit of a detector.

Grid leak. A high resistance connected across the grid capacitor or between the grid and the cathode to provide a d-c path from grid to cathode and to limit the accumulation of charge on the grid.

Grid limiting. Limiting the positive grid voltage (minimum output voltage) of vacuum-tube circuit by means of a large series grid resistor.

Ground. A metallic connection with the earth to establish ground potential. Also, a common return to a point of zero r-f potential, such as the chassis of a receiver or a transmitter.

Half-wave rectification. The process of rectifying an alternating current wherein only one-half of the input cycle is passed and the other half is blocked by the action of the rectifier, thus producing pulsating direct current.

Hard tube. A high vacuum electronic tube.

Harmonic. An integral multiple of a fundamental frequency. (The second harmonic is twice the frequency of the fundamental or first harmonic.)

Harmonic distortion. Amplitude distortion.

Heater. The tube element used to indirectly heat a cathode.

Henry (h). The basic unit of inductance.

Helmholts coil. A variometer having horizontal and vertical balanced coil windings, used to vary the angle of phase difference between any two similar waveforms of the same frequency.

Heterodyne. To beat or mix two signals of different frequencies.

High-frequency resistance. The resistance presented to the flow of high-frequency current. *See* Skin effect.

Horn radiator. Any open-ended metallic device for concentrating energy from a waveguide and directing this energy into space.

Hysteresis. A lagging of the magnetic flux in a magnetic material behind the magnetizing force which is producing it.

Image frequency. An undesired signal capable of beating with the local oscillator signal of a superheterodyne receiver which produces a difference frequency within the bandwidth of the i-f channel.

Impedance (Z). The total opposition offered to the flow of an alternating current. It may consist of any combination of resistance, inductive reactance, and capacitive reactance.

Impedance coil. *See* Choke.

Impedance coupling. The use of a tuned circuit or an impedance coil as the common coupling element between two circuits.

Impulse. Any force acting over a comparatively short period of time, such as a momentary rise in voltage.

Indirectly heated cathode. A cathode which is brought to the temperature necessary for electron emission by a separate heater element. Compare *Directly heated cathode.*

Inductance (L). The property of a circuit which tends to oppose a change in the existing current.

Induction. The act or process of producing voltage by the relative motion of a magnetic field across a conductor.

Inductive reactance (X_1). The opposition to the flow of alternating or pulsating current caused by the inductance of a circuit. It is measured in ohms.

Inductor. A circuit element designed so that its inductance is its most important electrical property; a coil.

Infinite. Extending indefinitely; having innumerable parts, capable of endless division within itself.

In phase. Applied to the condition that exists when two waves of the same frequency pass through their maximum and minimum values of like polarity at the same instant.

Instantaneous value. The magnitude at any particular instant when a value is continually varying with respect to time.

Integrating circuit. A circuit which produces an output voltage substantially in proportion to the frequency and amplitude of the input voltage.

Intensify. To increase the brilliance of an image on the screen of a cathode-ray tube.

Intensity modulation. The control of the brilliance of the trace on the screen of a cathode-ray tube in conformity with the signal.

Interelectrode capacitance. The capacitance existing between the electrodes in a vacuum tube.

Intermediate frequency (i-f). The fixed frequency to which r-f carrier waves are converted in a superheterodyne receiver.

Inverse peak voltage. The highest instantaneous negative potential which the plate can acquire with respect to the cathode without danger of injuring the tube.

Ion. An elementary particle of matter or a small group of such particles having a net positive or negative charge.

Ionization. Process by which ions are produced in solids, liquids, or gases.

Ionization potential. The lowest potential at which ionization takes place within a gas-filled tube.

Ionosphere. A region composed of highly ionized layers of atmosphere from 70 to 250 miles above the surface of the earth.

Kilo (k). A prefix meaning 1,000.

Kilocycle (kc). One thousand cycles; conversationally used to indicate 1,000 cycles per second.

Klystron. A tube in which oscillations are generated by the bunching of electrons (that is, velocity modulation). This tube utilizes the transit time between two given electrodes to deliver pulsating energy to a cavity resonator in order to sustain oscillations within the cavity.

Lag. The amount one wave is behind another in time; expressed in electrical degrees.

Lead The opposite of *lag*. Also, a wire or connection.

Leakage. The electrical loss due to poor insulation.

Lecher line. A section of open-wire transmission line used for measurements of standing waves.

Limiting. Removal by electronic means of one or both extremities of a waveform at a predetermined level.

Linear. Having an output which varies in direct proportion to the input.

Line-balance converter. A device used at the end of a coaxial line to isolate the outer conductor from ground.

Load. The impedance to which energy is being supplied.

Local oscillator. The oscillator used in a superheterodyne receiver the output of which is mixed with the desired r-f carrier to form the intermediate frequency.

Loose coupling. Less than critical coupling; coupling providing little transfer of energy.

Magnetic circuit. The complete path of magnetic lines of force.

Magnetic field (H). The space in which a magnetic force exists.

Magnetron. A vacuum-tube oscillator containing two electrodes, in which the flow of electrons from cathode to anode is controlled by an externally applied magnetic field.

Matched impedance. The condition which exists when two coupled circuits are so adjusted that their impedances are equal.

Meg (mega) (m). A prefix meaning one million.

Megacycle (M_c). One million cycles. Used conversationally to mean 1,000,000 cycles per second.

Metallic insulator. A shorted quarter-wave section of a transmission line which acts as an electrical insulator at a frequency corresponding to its quarter-wave length.

Mho. The unit of conductance.

Micro (μ). A prefix meaning one-millionth.

Microsecond (μs). One-millionth of a second.

Milli (m). A prefix meaning one-thousandth.

Milliampera (ma). One-thousandth of an ampere.

Mixer. A vacuum tube or crystal and suitable circuit used to combine the incoming and local-oscillator frequencies to produce an intermediate frequency. *See* Beat frequency.

Modulation. The process of varying the amplitude (amplitude modulation), the frequency (frequency modulation), or the phase (phase modulation) of a carrier wave in accordance with other signals in order to convey intelligence. The modulating signal may be an audiofrequency signal, video signal (as in television), or electrical pulses or tones to operate relays, etc.

Modulator. The circuit which provides the signal that varies the ampli- tude, frequency, or phase of the oscillations generated in the transmitter tube.

Multielectrode tube. A vacuum tube containing more than three electrodes associated with a single electron stream.

Multiunit tube. A vacuum tube containing within one envelope two or more groups of electrodes, each associated with separate electron streams.

Multivibrator. A type of relaxation oscillator for the generation of nonsinusoidal waves in which the output of each of its two tubes is coupled to the input of the other to sustain oscillations.

Mutual conductance (g_m). *See* Transconductance.

Mutual inductance. A circuit property existing when the relative position of two inductors causes the magnetic lines of force from one to link with the turns of the other.

Negative feedback. *See* Degeneration.

Neon bulb. A glass bulb containing two electrodes in neon gas at low pressure.

Network. Any electrical circuit containing two or more interconnected elements.

Neutralisation. The process of nullifying the voltage fed back through the interelectrode capacitance of an amplifier tube, by providing an equal voltage of opposite phase; generally necessary only with triode tubes.

Node. A zero point; specifically, a current node is a point of zero current and a voltage node is a point of zero voltage.

Noninductive capacitor. A capacitor in which the inductive effects at high frequencies are reduced to the minimum.

Noninductive circuit. A circuit in which inductance is reduced to a minimum or negligible value.

Nonlinear. Having an output which does not vary in direct proportion to the input.

Ohm (ω). The unit of electrical resistance.

Open circuit. A circuit which does not provide a complete path for the flow of current.

Optimum coupling. See Critical coupling.

Oscillator. A circuit capable of converting direct current into alternating current of a frequency determined by the constants of the circuit. It generally uses a vacuum tube.

Oscillatory circuit. A circuit in which oscillations can be generated or sustained.

Oscillograph. See Oscilloscope.

Oscilloscope. An instrument for showing, visually, graphical representations of the waveforms encountered in electrical circuits.

Overdriven amplifier. An amplifier designed to distort the input signal waveform by a combination of cut-off limiting and saturation limiting.

Overload. A load greater than the rated load of an electrical device.

Parallel feed. Application of a d-c voltage to the plate or grid of a tube in parallel with an a-c circuit so that the d-c and a-c components flow in separate paths. Also called shunt feed.

Parallel-resonant circuit. A resonant circuit in which the applied voltage is connected across a parallel circuit formed by a capacitor and an inductor.

Paraphase amplifier. An amplifier which converts a single input into a push-pull output.

Parasitic suppressor. A resistor in a vacuum-tube circuit to prevent un-wanted oscillations.

Peaking circuit. A type of circuit which converts an input to a peaked output waveform.

Peak plate current. The maximum instantaneous plate current passing through a tube.

Peak value. The maximum instantaneous value of a varying current, voltage, or power. It is equal to 1.414 times the effective value of a sine wave.

Pentode. A five-electrode vacuum tube containing a cathode, control, grid, screen grid, suppressor grid, and plate.

Phase difference. The time in electrical degrees by which one wave leads or lags another.

Phase inversion. A phase difference of 180 between two similar waveshapes of the same frequency.

Phase-splitting circuit. A circuit which produces from the same input waveform two output waveforms which differ in phase from each other.

Phosphorescence. The property of emitting light for some time after excitation by electronic bombardment.

Piezoelectric effect. The effect of producing a voltage by placing a stress, either by compression, by expansion, or by twisting, on a crystal, and, conversely, the effect of producing a stress in a crystal by applying a voltage to it.

Plate (P). The principal electrode in a tube to which the electron stream is attracted. See Anode.

Plate circuit. The complete electrical circuit connecting the cathode and plate of a vacuum tube.

Plate current (i_p). The current flowing in the plate circuit of a vacuum tube.

Plate detection. The operation of a vacuum-tube detector at or near cutoff so that the input signal is rectified in the plate circuit.

Plate dissipation. The power in watts consumed at the plate in the form of heat.

Plate efficiency. The ratio of the a-c power output from a tube to the average d-c power supplied to the plate circuit.

Plate impedance. See Plate resistance.

Plate-load impedance (R_L or Z_L). The impedance in the plate circuit across which the output signal voltage is developed by the alternating component of the plate current.

Plate modulation. Amplitude modulation of a class-C r-f amplifier by varying the plate voltage in accordance with the signal.

Plate resistance (r_p). The internal resistance to

the flow of alternating current between the cathode and plate of tube. It is equal to a small change in plate voltage divided by the corresponding change in plate current, and is expressed in ohms. It is also called a-c resistance, internal impedance, plate impedance, and dynamic plate impedance. The static plate resistance, or resistance to the flow of *direct current* is a different value. It is denoted by R_p.

Positive feedback. See Regeneration.

Potentiometer. A variable voltage divider; a resistor which has a variable contact arm so that any portion of the potential applied between its ends may be selected.

Power. The rate of doing work or the rate of expending energy. The unit of electrical power is the watt.

Power amplification. The process of amlifying a signal to produce a gain in power, as distinguished from voltage amplification. The gain in the ratio of the alternating power output to the alternating power input of an amplifier.

Power factor. The ratio of the actual power of an alternating or pulsating current, as measured by a wattmeter, to the apparent power, as indicated by ammeter and voltmeter readings. The power factor if an inductor, capacitor, or insulator is an expression of the losses.

Power tube. A vacuum tube designed to handle a greater amount of power than the ordinary voltage-amplifying tube.

Primary circuit. The first, in electrical order, of two or more coupled circuits, in which a change in current induces a voltage in the other or secondary circuits; such as the primary winding of a transformer.

Propagation. See Wave propagation.

Pulsating current. A unidirectional current which increases and decreases in magnitude.

Push-pull circuit. A push-pull circuit usually refers to an amplifier circuit using two vacuum tubes in such a fashion that when one vacuum tube is operating on a positive alternation, the other vacuum tube operates on a negative alternation.

Q. The figure of merit of efficiency of a circuit or coil. Numerically it is equal to the inductive reactance divided by the resistance of the circuit or coil.

Radiate. To send out energy, such as r-f waves, into space.

Radiation resistance. A fictitious resistance which may be considered to dissipate the energy radiated from the antenna.

Radio frequency (r-f). Any frequency of electrical energy capable of propagation into space. Radio frequencies normally are much higher than sound-wave frequencies.

Radio-frequency amplification. The amplification of a radio wave by a receiver before detection, or by a transmitter before radiation.

Radio-frequency choke (RFC). An air-core or powdered iron core coil used to impede the flow of r-f currents.

Radio-frequency component. See Carrier.

Ratio. The value obtained by dividing one number by another, indicating their relative proportions.

Reactance (X). The opposition offered to the flow of an alternating current by the inductance, capacitance, or both, in any circuit.

Reciprocal. The value obtained by dividing the number 1 by any quantity.

Rectifier. A device used to change alternating current to unidirectional current.

Reflected impedance. See Coupled impedance.

Reflection. The turning back of a radio wave caused by reradiation from any conducting surface which is large in comparison to the wavelength of the radio wave.

Reflector. A metallic object placed behind a radiating antenna to prevent r-f radiation in an undesired direction and to reinforce radiation in a desired direction.

Regeneration. The process of returning a part of the output signal of an amplifier to its input circuit in such a manner that it reinforces the grid excitation and thereby increases the total amplification.

Regulation (voltage). The ratio of the change in voltage due to a load to the open-circuit voltage, expressed in per cent.

Relaxation oscillator. A circuit for the generation of nonsinusoidal waves by gradually storing and quickly releasing energy either in the electric field of a capacitor or in the magnetic field of an inductor.

Reluctance. The opposition to magnetic flux.

Resistance (R). The opposition to the flow of current caused by the nature and physical dimensions of a conductor.

Resistor. A circuit element whose chief characteristic is resistance; used to oppose the flow of current.

Resonance. The condition existing in a circuit in which the inductive and capacitive reactances cancel.

Resonance curve. A graphical representation of the manner in which a resonant circuit responds to various frequencies at and near the resonant frequency.

Rheostat. A variable resistor.

Ripple voltage. The fluctuations in the output voltage of a rectifier, filter, or generator.

rms. Abbreviation of root mean square. See Effective value.

Saturation. The condition existing in any circuit when an increase in the driving signal produces no further change in the resultant effect.

Saturation limiting. Limiting the minimum output voltage of a vacuum-tube circuit by operating the tube in the region of plate-current saturation (not to be confused with emission saturation).

Saturation point. The point beyond which an increase in either grid voltage, plate voltage, or both produces no increase in the existing plate current.

Screen dissipation. The power dissipated in the form of heat on the screen grid as the result of bombardment by the electron stream.

Screen grid (S_c). An electrode placed between the control grid and the plate of a vacuum tube to reduce interelectrode capacitance.

Secondary. The output coil of a transformer. See Primary circuit.

Secondary emission. The emission of electrons knocked loose from the plate, grid, or fluorescent screen of a vacuum tube by the impact or bombardment of electrons arriving from the cathode.

Selectivity. The degree to which a receiver is capable of discriminating between signals of different carrier frequencies.

Self-bias. The bias of a tube created by the voltage drop developed across a resistor through which either its cathode current or its grid current flows.

Self-excited oscillator. An oscillator depending on its resonant circuits for frequency determination. See Crystal oscillator.

Self-induction. The production of a counter-electromotive force in a conductor when its own magnetic field collapses or expands with a change in current in the conductor.

Sensitivity. The degree of response of a circuit to signals of the frequency to which it is tuned.

Series feed. Application of the d-c voltage to the plate or grid of a tube through the same impedance in which the alternating current flows. Compare *Parallel feed.*

Series resonance. The condition existing in a circuit when the source of voltage is in series with an inductor and capacitor whose reactances cancel each other at the applied frequency and thus reduce the impedance to a minimum.

Series-resonant circuit. A resonant circuit in which the capacitor and the inductor are in series with the applied voltage.

Shielding. A metallic covering used to prevent magnetic or electrostatic coupling between adjacent circuits.

Short-circuit. A low-impedance or zero-impedance path between two points.

Shunt. Parallel. A parallel resistor placed in an ammeter to increase its range.

Shunt feed. See Parallel feed. *Sine wave.* The curve traced by the projection on a uniform time scale of the end of a rotating arm, or vector. Also known as a sinusoidal wave.

Skin effect. The tendency of alternating currents to flow near the surface of a conductor, thus being restricted to a small part of the total cross-sectional area. This effect increases the resistance and becomes more marked as the frequency rises.

Soft tube. A vacuum tube the characteristics of which are adversely affected by the presence of gas in the tube; not to be confused with tubes designed to operate with gas inside them.

Solenoid. A multiturn coil of wire wound in a

uniform layer or layerson a hollow cylindrical form.

Space charge. The cloud of electrons existing in the space between the cathode and plate in a vacuum tube, formed by the electrons emitted from the cathode in excess of those immediately attracted to the plate.

Space current. The total current flowing between the cathode and all the other electrodes in a tube. This includes the plate current, grid current, screen-grid current, and any other electrode current which may be present.

Stability. Freedom from undesired variation.

Standing wave. A distribution of current and voltage on a transmission line formed by two sets of waves traveling in opposite directions, and characterized by the presence of a number of points of successive maxima and minima in the distribution curves.

Static. A fixed nonvarying condition; without motion.

Static characteristics. The characteristics of a tube with no output load and with d-c potentials applied to the grid and plate.

Superheterodyne. A receiver in which the incoming signal is mixed with a locally generated signal to produce a predetermined intermediate frequency.

Suppressor grid (Su). An electrode used in a vacuum tube to minimize the harmful effects of secondary emission from the plate.

Surge. Sudden changes of current or voltage in a circuit.

Surge impedance (Co). See Characteristic impedance.

Sweep circuit. The part of a cathode-ray oscilloscope which provides a time-reference base.

Swing. The variation in frequency or amplitude of an electrical quantity.

Swinging choke. A choke with an effective inductance which varies with the amount of current passing through it. It is used in some power-supply filter circuits.

Synchronous. Happening at the same time; having the same period and phase.

Tank circuit. See Parallel-resonant circuit.

Tetrode. A four-electrode vacuum tube containing a cathode, control grid, screen grid, and plate.

Thermionic emission. Electron emission caused by heating an emitter.

Thermocouple ammeter. An ammeter which operates by means of a voltage produced by the heating effect of a current passed through the junction of two dissimilar metals. It is used for r-f measurements.

Thyratron. A hot-cathode, gas-discharge tube in which one or more electrodes are used to control electrostatically the starting of an unidirectional flow of current.

Tight coupling. Degree of coupling in which practically all of the magnetic lines of force produced by one coil link a second coil.

Trace. A visible line or lines appearing on the screen of a cathode-ray tube in operation.

Transconductance (G_m). The ratio of the change in plate current to the change in grid voltage producing this change in plate current, while all other electrode voltages remain constant.

Transformer. A device composed of two or more coils, linked by magnetic lines of force, used to transfer energy from one circuit to another.

Transient. The voltage or current which exists as the result of a change from one steady-state condition to another.

Transit time. The time which electrons take to travel between the cathode and the plate of a vacuum tube.

Transmission lines. Any conductor or system of conductors used to carry electrical energy from its source to a load.

Triggering. Starting an action in another circuit, which then functions for a time under its own control.

Triode. A three-electrode vacuum tube, containing a cathode, control grid, and plate.

Tuned circuit. A resonant circuit.

Tuning. The process of adjusting a radio circuit so that it resonates at the desired frequency.

Unbalanced line. A transmission line in which the voltages on the two conductors are not equal with respect to ground; for example, a coaxial line.

Unidirectional. In one direction only.

Vacuum-tube voltmeter (VTVM). A device which uses either the amplifier characteristic or the rectifier characteristic of a vacuum tube or both to measure either d-c or a-c voltages. Its input impedance is very high, and the current used to actuate the meter movement is not taken from the circuit being measured. It can be used to obtain accurate measurements in sensitive circuits.

Variable-u tube. A vacuum tube in which the control grid is irregularly spaced, so that the grid exercises a different amount of control on the electron stream at different points within its operating range.

Variocoupler. Two independent inductors, so arranged mechanically that their mutual inductance (coupling) can be varied.

Variometer. A variocoupler having its two coils connected in series, and so mounted that the movable coil may be rotated within the fixed coil, thus changing the total inductance of the unit.

Vector. A line used to represent both direction and magnitude.

Velocity modulation. A method of modulation in which the input signal voltage is used to change the velocity of electrons in a constant-current electron beam so that the electrons are grouped into bunches.

Video amplifier. A circuit capable of amplifying a very wide range of frequencies, including and exceeding the audio band of frequencies.

Volt (V). The unit of electrical potential.

Voltage amplification. The process of amplifying a signal to produce a gain in voltage. The voltage gain of an amplifier is the ratio of its alternating-voltage output to its alternating-voltage input.

Voltage divider. An impedance connected across a voltage source. The load is connected across a fraction of this impedance so that the load voltage is substantially in proportion to this fraction.

Voltage doubter. A method of increasing the voltage by rectifying both halves of a cycle and causing the outputs of both halves to be additive.

Voltage regulation. A measure of the degree to which a power source maintains its output-voltage stability under varying load conditions.

Watt (w). The unit of electrical power.

Wave. Loosely, an electromagnetic impulse, periodically changing in intensity and traveling through space. More specifically, the graphical representation of the intensity of that impulse over a oeriod of time.

Waveform. The shape of the wave obtained when instantaneous values of an a-c quantity are plotted against time in rectangular coordinates.

Wavelength (A). The distance, usually expressed in meters, traveled by a wave during the time interval of one complete cycle. It is equal to the velocity divided by the frequency.

Wave propagation. The transmission of r-f energy through space.

Wien-bridge circuit. A circuit in which the various values of capacitance and resistance are made to balance with each other at a certain frequency.

X. The symbol for reactance.

Z. The symbol for impedance.

ELECTRONICS SYMBOLS

AMPLIFIER (2)

general
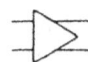

with two inputs
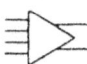

with two outputs

with adjustable gain
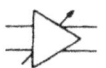

with associated power supply
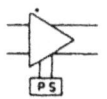

with associated attenuator
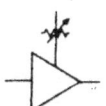

with external feedback path
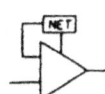

Amplifier Letter Combinations (amplifier-use identification in symbol if required)

BDG   Bridging
BST   Booster
CMP   Compression
DC   Direct Current
EXP   Expansion
LIM   Limiting
MON   Monitoring
PGM   Program
PRE   Preliminary
PWR   Power
TRQ   Torque

ANTENNA (3)

general

dipole

loop

counterpoise
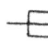

ARRESTER, LIGHTNING (4)

general
—•—

carbon block
—□□—

electrolytic or aluminum cell
—»»—

horn gap

protective gap

sphere gap

valve or film element

multigap

ATTENUATOR, FIXED (see PAD) (57)
(same symbol as variable attenuator, without variability)

ATTENUATOR, VARIABLE (5)

balanced
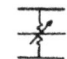

unbalanced

AUDIBLE SIGNALING DEVICE (6)

bell, electrical; ringer, telephone

buzzer

horn, electrical; loudspeaker; siren; underwater sound hydrophone, projector or transducer

Horn, Letter Combinations (if required)

*HN   Horn, electrical
*HW   Howler
*LS   Loudspeaker
*SN   Siren
‡EM   Electromagnetic with moving coil
‡EMN Electromagnetic with moving coil and neutralizing winding
‡MG   Magnetic armature
‡PM   Permanent magnet with moving coil

identification replaces (*) asterisk and (‡) dagger)

sounder, telegraph

BATTERY (7)

generalized direct current source; one cell

multicell

CAPACITOR (8)

general

polarized

adjustable or variable
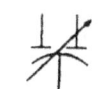

continuously adjustable or variable differential
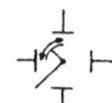

phase-shifter
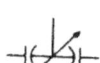

split-stator

feed-through

CELL, PHOTOSENSITIVE (Semiconductor) (9)

asymmetrical photoconductive transducer

symmetrical photoconductive transducer

ELECTRONICS SYMBOLS

photovoltaic transducer; solar cell

CIRCUIT BREAKER (11)

general

with magnetic overload

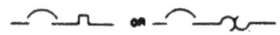

drawout type

CIRCUIT ELEMENT (12)

general

Circuit Element Letter Combinations (replaces (*) asterisk)

EG	Equalizer
FAX	Facsimile set
FL	Filter
FL-BE	Filter, band elimination
FL-BP	Filter, band pass
FL-HP	Filter, high pass
FL-LP	Filter, low pass
PS	Power supply
RG	Recording unit
RU	Reproducing unit
DIAL	Telephone dial
TEL	Telephone station
TPR	Teleprinter
TTY	Teletypewriter

Additional Letter Combinations (symbols preferred)

AR	Amplifier
AT	Attenuator
C	Capacitor
CB	Circuit breaker
HS	Handset
I	Indicating or switch board lamp
L	Inductor
J	Jack
LS	Loudspeaker
MIC	Microphone
OSC	Oscillator
PAD	Pad
P	Plug
HT	Receiver, headset
K	Relay
R	Resistor
S	Switch or key switch
T	Transformer
WR	Wall receptacle

CLUTCH; BRAKE (14)

disengaged when operating means is de-energized

engaged when operating means is de-energized

COIL, RELAY and OPERATING (16)

semicircular dot indicates inner end of wiring

CONNECTOR (18)

assembly, movable or stationary portion; jack, plug, or receptacle

jack or receptacle

plug

separable connectors

two-conductor switchboard jack

two-conductor switchboard plug

jacks normalled through one way

jacks normalled through both ways

2-conductor nonpolarized, female contacts

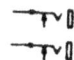

2-conductor polarized, male contacts

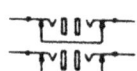

waveguide flange

plain, rectangular

choke, rectangular

engaged 4-conductor; the plug has 1 male and 3 female contacts, individual contact designations shown

coaxial, outside conductor shown carried through

coaxial, center conductor shown carried through; outside conductor not carried through

mated choke flanges in rectangular waveguide

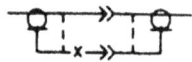

COUNTER, ELECTROMAGNETIC; MESSAGE REGISTER (26)

general

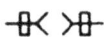

with a make contact

COUPLER, DIRECTIONAL (27)
(common coaxial/waveguide usage)

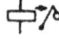

(common coaxial/waveguide usage)

E-plane aperture-coupling, 30-decibel transmission loss

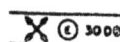

COUPLING (28)

by loop from coaxial to circular waveguide, direct-current grounds connected

CRYSTAL, PIEZO-ELECTRIC (62)

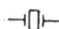

DELAY LINE (31)

general

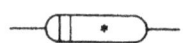

tapped delay

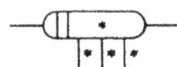

bifilar slow-wave structure (commonly used in traveling-wave tubes)

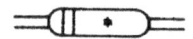

(length of delay indication replaces (*) asterisk)

DETECTOR, PRIMARY; MEASURING TRANSDUCER (30)
(see HALL GENERATOR and THERMAL CONVERTER)

DISCONTINUITY (33)
(common coaxial/waveguide usage)

equivalent series element, general

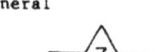

capacitive reactance

inductive reactance

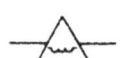

inductance-capacitance circuit, infinite reactance at resonance

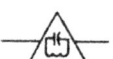

ELECTRONICS SYMBOLS

inductance-capacitance circuit, zero reactance at resonance

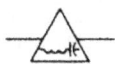

resistance

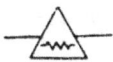

equivalent shunt element, general

capacitive susceptance

conductance

inductive susceptance

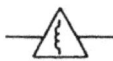

inductance-capacitance circuit, infinite susceptance at resonance

inductance-capacitance circuit, zero susceptance at resonance

ELECTRON TUBE (34)

triode

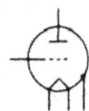

pentode, envelope connected to base terminal

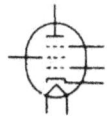

twin triode, equipotential cathode

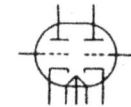

typical wiring figure to show tube symbols placed in any convenient position

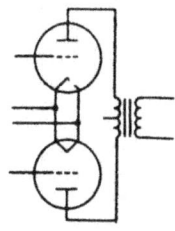

rectifier; voltage regulator (see LAMP, GLOW)

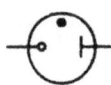

phototube, single and multiplier

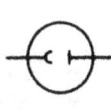 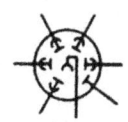

cathode-ray tube, electrostatic and magnetic deflection

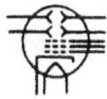 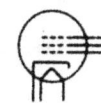

mercury-pool tube, ignitor and control grid (see RECTIFIER)

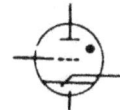

resonant magnetron, coaxial output and permanent magnet

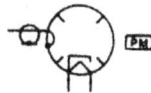

reflex klystron, integral cavity, aperture coupled

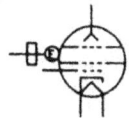

transmit-receive (TR) tube gas filled, tunable integral cavity, aperture coupled, with starter

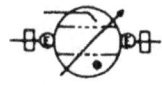

traveling-wave tube (typical)

forward-wave traveling-wave-tube amplifier shown with four grids, having slow-wave structure with attenuation, magnetic focusing by external permanent magnet, rf input and rf output coupling each E-plane aperture to external rectangular waveguide

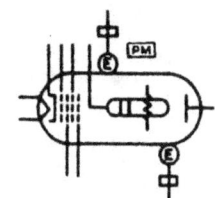

FERRITE DEVICES (100)

field polarization rotator

field polarization amplitude modulator

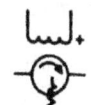

FUSE (36)

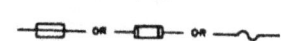

high-voltage primary cutout, dry

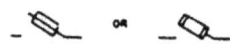

high-voltage primary cutout, oil

GOVERNOR (Contact-making) (37)

contacts shown here as closed

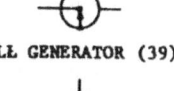

HALL GENERATOR (39)

HANDSET (40)

general

operator's set with push-to talk switch

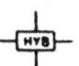

HYBRID (41)

general

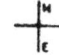

junction (common coaxial/waveguide usage)

circular

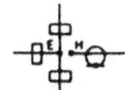

(E, H or HE transverse field indicators replace (*) asterisk)

rectangular waveguide and coaxial coupling

INDUCTOR (42)

general

ELECTRONICS SYMBOLS

magnetic core

tapped

adjustable, continuously adjustable

KEY, TELEGRAPH (43)

LAMP (44)

ballast lamp; ballast tube

lamp, fluorescent, 2 and 4 terminal

lamp, glow; neon lamp
a-c

d-c

lamp, incandescent

indicating lamp; switchboard lamp
(see VISUAL SIGNALING DEVICE)

LOGIC (see 806B and Y32-14)
(including some duplicate symbols; left and right-hand symbols are not mixed)

AND function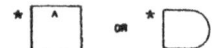

OR function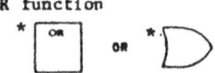

EXCLUSIVE-OR function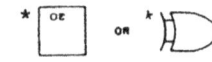

((*) input side of logic symbols in general)

condition indicators

state (logic negation)

O

a Logic Negation output becomes 1-state if and only if the input is not 1-state

an AND func. where output is low if and only if all inputs are high

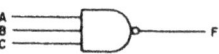

electric inverter

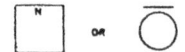

(elec. invtr. output becomes 1-state if and only if the input is 1-state) (elec. invtr. output is more pos. if and only if input is less pos.)

level (relative)

1-state is   1-state is
less +   more +

(symbol is a rt. triangle pointing in direction of flow)

an AND func. with input 1-states at more pos. level and output 1-state at less pos. level

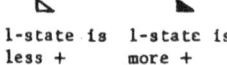

single shot (one output)

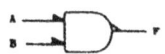

(waveform data replaces inside/outside (*))

schmitt trigger, waveform and two outputs

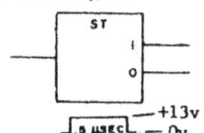

flip-flop, complementary

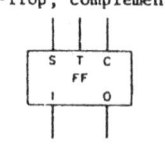

flip-flop, latch

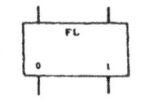

register

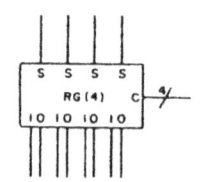

(binary register denoting four flip-flops and bits)

amplifier (see AMPLIFIER)

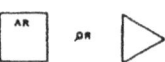

channel path(s) (see PATH, TRANSMISSION)

magnetic heads (see PICK-UP HEAD)

oscillator (see OSCILLATOR)

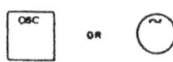

relay, contacts (see CONTACT, ELECTRICAL)
relay, electromagnetic (see RELAY COIL RECOGNITION)

signal flow (see DIRECTION OF FLOW)

time delay (see DELAY LINE)

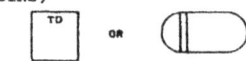

time delay with typical delay taps:

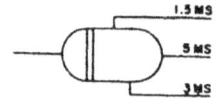

functions not otherwise symbolized

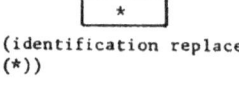

(identification replaces (*))

Logic Letter Combinations

S	set
C	clear (reset)
T	toggle (trigger)
(N)	number of bits
BO	blocking oscillator
CF	cathode follower
EF	emitter follower
FF	flip-flop
SS	single shot
ST	schmitt trigger
RG(N)	register (N stages)
SR	shift register

MACHINE, ROTATING (46)

generator

motor

METER, INSTRUMENT (48)

identification replaces (*) asterisk)

Meter Letter Combinations

A	Ammeter
AH	Ampere-hour
CMA	Contact-making (or breaking) ammeter
CMC	Contact-making (or breaking) clock
CMV	Contact-making (or breaking) voltmeter
CRO	Oscilloscope or cathode-ray oscillograph
DB	DB (decibel) meter
DBM	DBM (decibels referred to 1 milliwatt) meter
DM	Demand meter
DTR	Demand-totalizing relay
F	Frequency meter
G	Galvanometer
GD	Ground detector
I	Indicating
INT	Integrating
μA or UA	Microammeter
MA	Milliammeter
NM	Noise meter
OHM	Ohmmeter
OP	Oil pressure

ELECTRONICS SYMBOLS

MODE TRANSDUCER (53)

(common coaxial/waveguide usage)

transducer from rectangular waveguide to coaxial with mode suppression, direct-current grounds connected

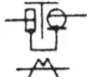

MOTION, MECHANICAL (54)

rotation applied to a resistor

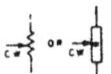

(identification replaces (*) asterisk)

NUCLEAR-RADIATION DETECTOR, gas filled; IONIZATION CHAMBER; PROPORTIONAL COUNTER TUBE; GEIGER-MULLER COUNTER TUBE (50) (see RADIATION-SENSITIVITY INDICATOR)

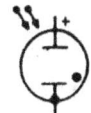

PATH, TRANSMISSION (58)

cable; 2-conductor, shield grounded and 5-conductor shielded

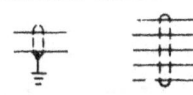

PICKUP HEAD (61)

general

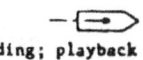

writing; recording

reading; playback

erasing

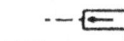

writing, reading, and erasing

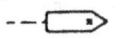

stereo

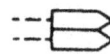

RECTIFIER (65)

semiconductor diode; metallic rectifier; electrolytic rectifier; asymmetrical varistor

mercury-pool tube power rectifier

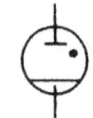

fullwave bridge-type

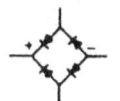

RESISTOR (68)

general

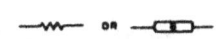

tapped

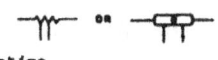

heating

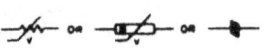

symmetrical varistor resistor, voltage sensitive (silicon carbide, etc.)

(identification marks replace (*) asterisk)

with adjustable contact

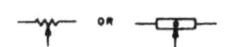

adjustable or continuously adjustable (variable)

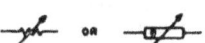

(identification replaces (*) asterisk)

RESONATOR, TUNED CAVITY (71)

(common coaxial/waveguide usage)

resonator with mode suppression coupled by an E-plane aperture to a guided transmission path and by a loop to a coaxial path

tunable resonator with direct-current ground connected to an electron device and adjustably coupled by an E-plane aperture to a rectangular waveguide

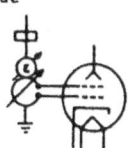

ROTARY JOINT, RF (COUPLER) (72)

general; with rectangular waveguide

(transmission path recognition symbol replaces (*) asterisk)

coaxial type in rectangular waveguide

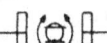

circular waveguide type in rectangular waveguide

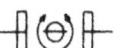

SEMICONDUCTOR DEVICE (73)
(Two Terminal, diode)

semiconductor diode; rectifier

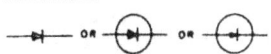

capacitive diode (also Varicap, Varactor, reactance diode, parametric diode)

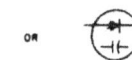

breakdown diode, unidirectional (also backward diode, avalanche diode, voltage regulator diode, Zener diode, voltage reference diode)

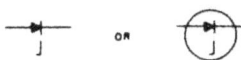

breakdown diode, bidirectional and backward diode (also bipolar voltage limiter)

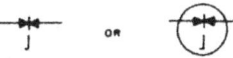

tunnel diode (also Esaki diode)

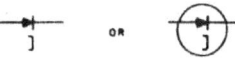

temperature-dependent diode

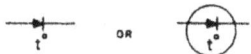

photodiode (also solar cell)

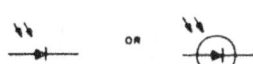

semiconductor diode, PNPN switch (also Shockley diode, four-layer diode and SCR).

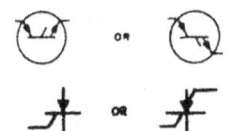

(Multi-Terminal, transistor, etc.)

PNP transistor

NPN transistor

unijunction transistor, N-type base

ELECTRONICS SYMBOLS

unijunction transistor, P-type base

field-effect transistor, N-type base

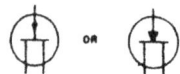

field-effect transistor, P-type base

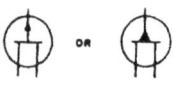

semiconductor triode, PNPN-type switch

semiconductor triode, NPNP-type switch

NPN transistor, transverse-biased base

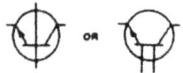

PNIP transistor, ohmic connection to the intrinsic region

NPIN transistor, ohmic connection to the intrinsic region

PNIN transistor, ohmic connection to the intrinsic region

NPIP transistor, ohmic connection to the intrinsic region

SQUIB (75)

explosive igniter

sensing link; fusible link operated

SWITCH (76)

push button, circuit closing (make)

push button, circuit opening (break)

nonlocking; momentary circuit closing (make)

nonlocking; momentary circuit opening (break)

transfer

locking, circuit closing (make)

locking, circuit opening (break)

transfer, 3-position

wafer

(example shown: 3-pole 3-circuit with 2 non-shorting and 1 shorting moving contacts)

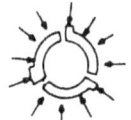

safety interlock, circuit opening and closing

2-pole field-discharge knife, with terminals and discharge resistor

(identification replaces (*) asterisk)

SYNCHRO (78)

Synchro Letter Combinations
CDX Control-differential transmitter
CT   Control transformer
CX   Control transmitter
TDR Torque-differential receiver
TDX Torque-differential transmitter
TR   Torque receiver
TX   Torque transmitter
RS   Resolver
B   Outer winding rotatable in bearings

THERMAL ELEMENT (83)

actuating device

thermal cutout; flasher

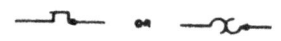

thermal relay

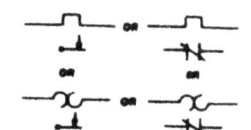

thermostat (operates on rising temperature), contact)

thermostat, make contact

thermostat, integral heater and transfer contacts

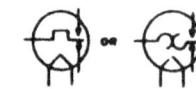

THERMISTOR; THERMAL RESISTOR (84)

with integral heater

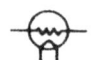

THERMOCOUPLE (85)

temperature-measuring

current-measuring, integral heater connected

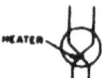

current-measuring, integral heater insulated

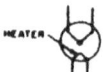

temperature-measuring, semiconductor

current-measuring, semiconductor

TRANSFORMER (86)

general

magnetic-core

one winding with adjustable inductance

separately adjustable inductance

adjustable mutual inductor, constant-current

ELECTRONICS SYMBOLS

autotransformer, 1-phase adjustable

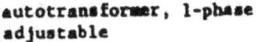

current, with polarity marking

potential, with polarity mark

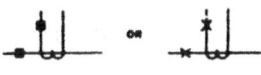

with direct-current connections and mode suppression between two rectangular waveguides

(common coaxial/waveguide usage)

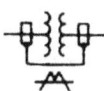

shielded, with magnetic core

with a shield between windings, connected to the frame

VIBRATOR; INTERRUPTER (87)

typical shunt drive (terminals shown)

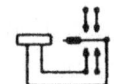

typical separate drive (terminals shown)

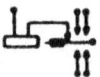

VISUAL SIGNALING DEVICE (88)

communication switchboard-type lamp

⊸◐

indicating, pilot, signaling, or switchboard light (see LAMP)

▭ or ⇨ or ⊙

(identification replaces (*) asterisk)

indicating light letter combinations

A   Amber
B   Blue
C   Clear
G   Green
NE Neon
O   Orange
OP Opalescent
P   Purple
R   Red
W   White
Y   Yellow

jeweled signal light

⊕

TRANSISTOR SYMBOLS

<u>Semiconductor, General</u>
BV .... Breakdown voltage
TA .... Ambient temperature
T_{ep} .... Operating temperature

<u>Transistor</u>
B, b .... Base electrode
C, c .... Collector electrode
C_{ib} .... Input capacitance (common base)
C_{ie} .... Input capacitance (common emitter)
C_{ob} .... Output capacitance (common base)
C_{oe} .... Output capacitance (common emitter)
E, e .... Emitter electrode
I_B .... Base current (dc)
i_b .... Base current (instantaneous)
I_C .... Collector current (dc)
i_c .... Collector current (instantaneous)
I_{CBO} .... Collector cutoff current (dc) emitter open

I_{CEO} .... Collector cutoff current (dc) base open
I_E .... Emitter current
R_B .... External base resistance
$r_{b'}$ .... Base spreading resistance
r_i .... Input junction resistance
V_{BB} .... Base supply voltage
V_c .... Collector voltage (with respect to ground or common point)
V_{BE} .... Base to emitter voltage (dc)
V_{CB} .... Collector to base voltage (dc)
V_{CE} .... Collector to emitter voltage (dc)
V_{ce} .... Collector to emitter voltage (rms)
v_{ce} .... Collector to emitter voltage (instantaneous)
V_{CE}(sat) .... Collector to emitter saturation voltage
V_{EBO} .... Emitter to base voltage (static)
V_{CC} .... Collector supply voltage
V_{EE} .... Emitter supply voltage

TUBE SYMBOLS

A_{hf}	High frequency gain
A_{lf}	Low frequency gain
A_v	Voltage gain
C_c	Coupling capacitor
C_d	Distributed capacitance
C_{gk}	Grid-to-cathode capacitance
C_{gp}	Grid-to-plate capacitance
C_i	Input capacitance
C_K	Cathode bypass capacitor
C_O	Output capacitance
C_{pk}	Plate-to-cathode capacitance
C_s	Shunt capacitance ($C_d + C_i + C_o$)
E_b	Plate volts (dc)
E_{bb}	Supply volts (dc)
E_{bo}	Quiescent plate voltage
E_{c1}	Control grid voltage
E_{c2}	Screen grid voltage
E_{cc}	Control grid supply voltage
E_f	Filament terminal voltage
e_b	Instantaneous total plate volts (ac and dc)
e_{c1}	Instantaneous total control grid volts (ac and dc)
e_{c2}	Instantaneous total screen grid volts (ac and dc)
e_{g1}	Instantaneous value of ac control grid volts
e_{g2}	Instantaneous value of ac screen grid volts
e_{po}	Instantaneous value of plate voltage above and below the quiescent value
E_g	RMS value of grid volts
E_p	RMS value of plate volts
g_m	Grid-plate transconductance (mutual conductance)
I_b	DC value of plate volts
I_{bo}	Quiescent value of plate current
I_{c1}	DC value of control grid current
I_{C2}	DC value of screen grid current
I_f	Filament or heater current
I_{g1}	RMS value of control grid current
I_{g2}	RMS value of screen grid current
I_{gml}	Crest values of ac current control grid
g_{m2}	Crest values of ac current screen grid
I_p	RMS' values of plate current
I_{pm}	Crest value of plate current
I_s	Total electron emission
i_b	Instantaneous total value of plate current
i_{c1}	Instantaneous total value of control grid current
i_{c2}	Instantaneous total value of screen grid current
i_{g1}	Instantaneous ac value of control grid current
i_{g2}	Instantaneous ac value of screen grid current
i_p	Instantaneous ac value of plate current
i_{po}	Instantaneous values of plate current above and below the uiescent value
R_b	DC plate resistance
R_g	DC grid resistance
R_k	DC cathode resistance
R_L	Plate load resistance
r_p	AC plate resistance
μ	Amplification factor

www.ingramcontent.com/pod-product-compliance
Lightning Source LLC
Chambersburg PA
CBHW081822300426
44116CB00014B/2455